PERSONAL
COLOR

PERSONAL

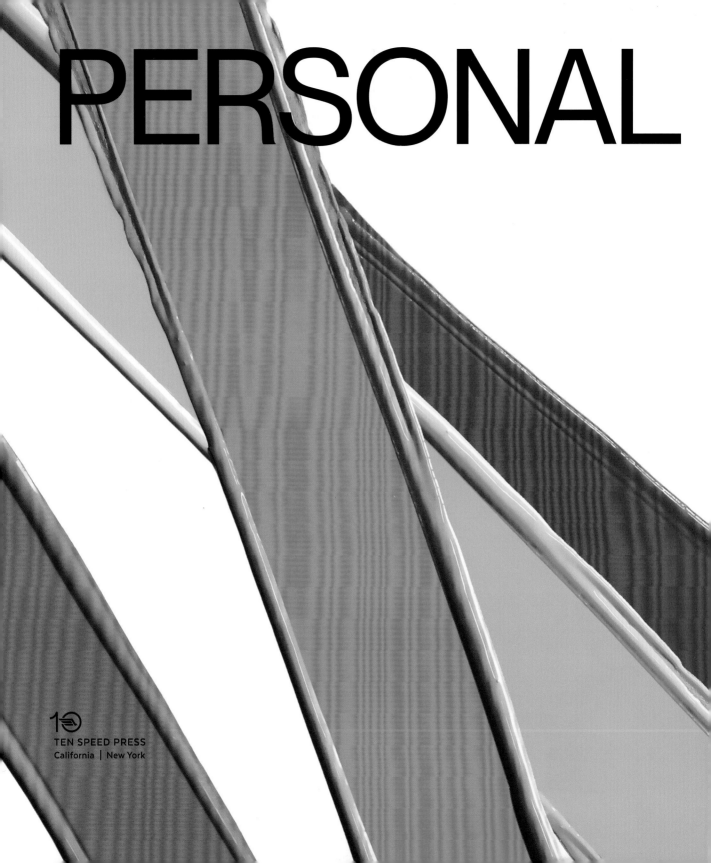

TEN SPEED PRESS
California | New York

COLOR

The Definitive Guide to Finding
and Wearing Your Best Colors

ANUSCHKA REES

Contents

Part 1
COLOR THEORY

Part 2
FIND YOUR SEASON

Part 3
YOUR COLORS

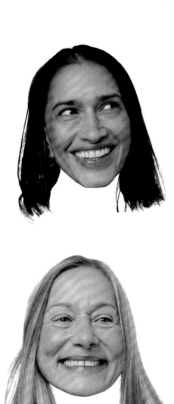
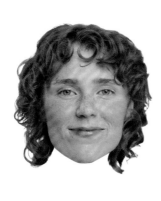
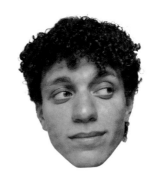
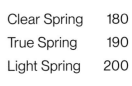

Clear Spring   180
True Spring   190
Light Spring   200

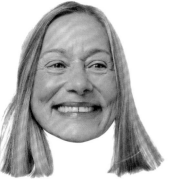
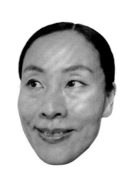
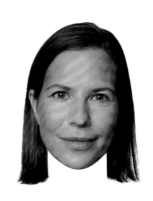

Light Summer   210
True Summer   220
Soft Summer   230

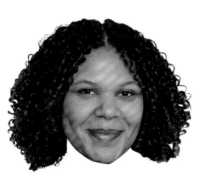
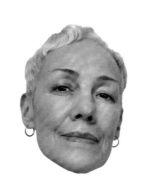
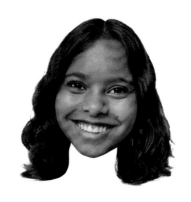

Soft Autumn   240
True Autumn   250
Deep Autumn   260

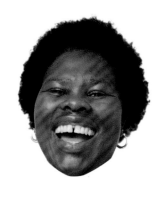
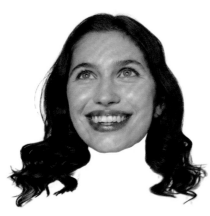
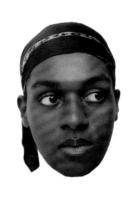

Deep Winter   270
True Winter   280
Clear Winter   290

INTRODUCTION

Why Some Colors Look Better on You Than Others

If you've ever gotten dressed and ready to go out with friends, or shared clothes with someone, you know that the same color can look striking on one person but off on another. The same exact shade can make one person look fresh and glowy—like they've just spent a week at a luxe Mediterranean wellness resort—but completely wash out another.

Have you ever wondered why that is? Why does your friend's charcoal coat look so chic on her but all shades of dull on you? Why can some people pull off bright crimson lipstick on a Tuesday, while others look borderline clownlike after a second layer of tinted lip balm?

The answer is: color theory. Or, more specifically, color harmony.

Color theory is the art and science of colors—their properties, how they can be mixed, and how we perceive them. Color harmony is a key field within color theory that explores why to the human eye certain shades look better together than others. The principles of color theory and color harmony are used by artists, designers, and other creatives around the world. Illustrators use them to select a palette for their artwork, filmmakers to calibrate the mood of their scenes, and art directors to create eye-catching ads for their clients.

Do not mistake the principles of color harmony for societal beauty standards. They were not created by corporations and are not inherently rooted in sexist gender roles. Like many other design principles,

GLOSSARY
Color theory

Color theory is the study of color: its attributes, how we perceive it, and how to measure and utilize it. It encompasses a range of fields, including color harmony, color mixing, color symbolism, and color psychology.

such as symmetry and balance, they were often discovered by artists who studied natural phenomena to figure out what makes them so aesthetically pleasing—and how to re-create that effect in their work.

Chances are, you are already using aspects of color theory in your everyday life. When you pick up flowers from the farmers' market, for example, and try to imagine which ones will look best on your kitchen counters. When you dial up the saturation and contrast of your pics before posting them on social media or sending them to someone. When you use peach-hued concealer to correct circles under your eyes, and even when you're adjusting the brightness level of your computer screen. All involve principles of color theory (how colors work) and color harmony (how two or more shades look next to each other).

And in this book, we'll use those same principles to figure out which shades best accentuate your unique color essence. What you do with this information is up to you: Self-expression and personal taste always trump color harmony. Use this book to explore the world of color and experiment just like artists do—color theory is just one of many creative tools in their tool belt.

GLOSSARY
Color harmony

Color harmony is a field within color theory that explores why certain shade combinations will be visually appealing to the human eye.

What is color analysis?

Color analysis is a framework that shows people which shades best harmonize with their skin tone, hair, and eyes. It was popularized in the 1980s by the mega-bestseller *Color Me Beautiful,* written by stylist and image consultant Carole Jackson. The book introduced four types: Spring, Summer, Autumn, and Winter, and recommended a different palette for each. Whether Carole Jackson really was the first to come up with the system has been the subject of debate. Some credit Hollywood stylist Suzanne Caygill, who is said to have created custom palettes for her clients that were named after seasons starting in the 1950s.

But the idea that one's complexion, hair, and eyes have an influence on the colors that suit them precedes Caygill too: In 1928, for example, a little booklet titled *Charts of Becoming Colors* featuring "correct and fashionable colors" was all the rage. Artists also began using seasons to characterize palettes long before *Color Me Beautiful* hit the scene. Derived from the hues of landscapes (in the Northern Hemisphere), fall tends to be associated with warm and earthy colors and winter with icy, cool shades. Spring is characterized by delicate shades of blossoming flowers, and summer by either vibrant brights or the softer pastels of a hazy summer's day.

As a millennial, I was not around for the original craze surrounding color analysis, but my mom—a fashion-conscious twentysomething at the time—was part of the generation whose entire approach to fashion and beauty was shaped by terms and concepts from *Color Me Beautiful*.

I had heard my mom use seasons as adjectives before ("that's a Winter blue"), but it wasn't until I found myself in a major preteen crisis that I came to understand what she was talking about. It was the early aughts and, for a few months, no self-respecting eighth grader would come to school without black eyeliner and flat-ironed hair. I had the hair part down but could not understand why all of my friends looked so incredibly cool with their kohl-rimmed eyes while I looked like a ghost child with Sharpie on her face. One day—after I requested to dig into her stash of makeup since my liners "weren't working"—my mom said, "Well, of course black's not going to suit you, you're a Spring type." She eventually handed me a worn paperback that had loose pages poking out and notes scribbled all over the margins. And so I was introduced to the great big world of seasonal color analysis.

Since the 1980s, a lot has happened in that world: *Color Me Beautiful* expanded its framework from four to twelve seasons, and social media introduced millions of people to color analysis. That renewed popularity has muddied the waters quite a bit. The sheer wealth of often conflicting information can make the whole concept seem incredibly complex, when, in reality, it's quite simple.

TRUE OR FALSE?
The right color can help you balance out and correct your undertone.

False! Color analysis is about leaning into your natural color essence. We are not trying to correct, fix, or balance out anything, because your natural coloring is already perfectly harmonious as it is.

Why is there so much conflicting information in the first place? Because color analysis originated at a time when expert knowledge (and expert status) was still very much king, and people were used to trusting professional advice. A product of its time, *Color Me Beautiful* is prescriptive without ever revealing its formula: Readers are told how to find their season and which colors to wear, but Carole Jackson never explains why that palette supposedly suits them—or, really, much else. Without a clear formula or framework for readers to refer back to, it's no wonder that over time people have filled in the gaps themselves with a mix of misconceptions, outdated fashion rules, and general style advice.

Now, it's not at all a bad thing that concepts develop over time or even branch out into something completely different. Some color analysts work with sixteen, twenty-four, or even thirty-six seasons. Some take into account your style, your personality, or your aura. As long as you know what the advice you are getting is based on, no system of color analysis is more or less valid than another.

TRUE OR FALSE?
When you get older, you should stop wearing bold colors.

Says who? It's true that most people's coloring changes over time, and your best colors at thirty-five may not be exactly the same as your best colors at seventy-five. It's also true that most people will favor slightly more muted and less intense tones as they age. However, depending on your baseline, a "slightly more muted" shade could mean a saturated flamingo pink or a vivid French blue. Whether you shine in bold brights or in a gentler palette depends on your unique color essence–age is irrelevant.

Key ideas of modern color analysis

In this book, every piece of advice is firmly rooted in fundamental color theory and the principles of color harmony. Color harmony is universal and independent of trends, cultural norms, and personal taste.

A core premise of color harmony is that your body already comes with a pre-installed color palette that is innately harmonious and aesthetic. Your skin tone, hair color, and eye color perfectly harmonize with one another. Why? Because your natural coloring came into existence organically and so, like most things in nature, already follows the universal principles of color harmony. Carole Jackson put it like this: "Nature is the most brilliant designer of all!"

A consequence of this premise is that color harmony is not corrective. We are not trying to improve, balance out, or fix anything. At no point will I tell you what to wear to get closer to any sort of ideal, because there is no one ideal. We all have a unique color essence that we can choose to lean in to, embrace, and accentuate.

Shades that honor that essence will look radiant and effortless on you. People will notice your face before they notice your outfit. Of course, it's entirely possible that sometimes you may not want that. Sometimes you may not want to look harmonious—you want to make a statement.

Many people consider neutrals a "safe" choice, but almost all neutrals are actually quite extreme from a color standpoint and ironically harder to pull off than many other colors.

Compare the two color palettes above. Can you see how, in the second palette, one of the swatches sticks out? The same happens when you wear a shade that is the opposite of your coloring. It's a little jarring and seems extra bold and dressed up on you, while it may look totally natural on someone with different coloring. But does it look "bad"? No! No color will make you look unattractive. The last thing I want is for you to end up with a mental list of colors that you are "not allowed" to wear. My goal is that, after reading this book, you'll end up wearing a broader range of colors than ever before. I want to give you the confidence to go beyond neutrals and whatever shades are currently on-trend or considered safe and to start exploring hues you had never even considered. Perhaps you've always been convinced that all shades of pink look terrible on you. But pink is a huge category that includes an infinite number of shades that can look very different. Maybe you don't love a bright Barbie pink on yourself, but what about a dusty mauve or a rich boysenberry? Let's not cut out entire hue families from our sartorial diet just yet!

As you dive into this book, I invite you to set aside any existing beliefs you may have about your coloring and look at it with fresh eyes. Throughout your life you will have inevitably picked up all sorts of miscellaneous chatter about the types of colors that suit you: Your skin is "white like a sheet," according to your aunt; you look "stupid" in pink, according to your middle school bully, but "so chic" in cobalt blue, according to that guy at work. And maybe each one of these people was giving you accurate information from their point of view. But you can't be sure to what degree that point of view is based on color harmony, trends, or random associations that person has to specific colors. Perhaps a hairdresser recommended an "ashier shade of brown to complement your cool complexion," but then, apparently, your skin has a "warm-neutral undertone" if you go by your favorite foundation shade. Beauty professionals, brands, and even color analysts may have different definitions of what exactly constitutes a warm, cool, or olive skin tone. One color analyst may classify you as a Soft Autumn, another as a True Autumn because each defines the color seasons slightly differently. As long as the color palettes they recommend are adjusted to these definitions, neither of them is more correct than the other. For this book, I challenge you to start from scratch.

Before we continue, a disclaimer: Throughout this book, I will be referring to your "best colors" and discussing which shades "suit," "flatter," or "work for" you. All of these terms are simply short for "harmonizes with your coloring, according to color harmony." They do not refer to how attractive a shade will make you look. If I say you "can" wear a specific shade, I mean "this shade is a good choice if your aim is maximum color harmony, but of course, you can and should wear whatever you want."

TRUE OR FALSE?
You should only wear colors that are recommended for your type.

False! You should only wear colors that you want to wear. In this book, you'll learn which tones harmonize with your coloring, and which may clash a little. But what you do with that information is up to you. Color harmony is not mandatory.

How can color analysis work on all skin tones?

There is no way around the fact that color analysis has not worked equally well for all skin tones in the past. Even today, many of the available resources on color analysis employ a painfully Eurocentric approach that carefully distinguishes between "light ash blond" and "champagne blond" while typing the majority of people of color as one of two types out of twelve. This is because these approaches use the absolute value (light to deep) of someone's coloring as one of the three key variables that determine their season. In *Color Me Beautiful,* Carol Jackson even posits "medium-brown hair" as a midway reference point for this variable. In other words, anyone with hair deeper than medium-brown could only be typed as a Winter or Autumn, and anyone with deep brown or black hair would usually be deemed a Deep Autumn or Deep Winter.

But, of course, not everyone with dark brown or black hair is suited to the same colors. Some people of color look great in rich, high-intensity colors, while others shine in less intense, lighter shades. From the beginning, my two goals for this book have been: first, to develop a system of color analysis that is firmly rooted in fundamental color theory, and second, to make sure it caters to all skin tones. I quickly realized that reaching my first goal would also take care of the second: from a color theory perspective, there is absolutely no reason for any season to be Caucasian-only. In a color analysis system that fully aligns with color theory, all seasons are found across all ethnicities.

A note on the models featured in this book

Great effort went into making sure the photos in this book demystify the color analysis process for all readers, regardless of skin tone, ethnicity, or age. We photographed fifty people (a mix of friends, friends of friends, and professional models), yet even these fifty models couldn't come close to capturing the vast diversity of human coloring in this world. Because of this, it's highly likely that you will not find a person in this book whose coloring is precisely like your own in all aspects. In fact, I strongly caution against trying to find a perfect color twin among the models. Many aspects we use to describe people in everyday life (brunette, freckles, green eyes, Southeast Asian) matter little to not at all for color analysis. If you have bright red hair, you may be tempted to assume you are a True Spring, like Lena, the only red-haired model in the book. But based on hair color alone, you are equally as likely to be a Soft Autumn, True Autumn, or Light Spring. What makes Lena a True Spring is not her hair color but the combination of her hair color, skin tone, undertone, eye color, contrast level, and natural luminosity. So, rather than attempting to find your best match among the models, use the photos to fully understand all the different attributes of someone's coloring (like undertone and so on), then apply that knowledge to your own unique coloring.

The two rules of color impact

You can use your color season to choose colors for your clothes, hair, and makeup. You can even use it to pick a flattering background for photos, video calls, or social media content. But please don't worry about every bracelet, pair of shoes, or belt buckle. How much of a color you are wearing, and where on your body, matters. There are two rules you can use to gauge a color's impact:

Rule 1: The closer a color is to your face, the greater the impact.

Only colors that exist in the same visual field as your face have any real impact on overall color harmony. Roughly, that includes any item above your waistline, and the closer an item is to your face, the higher the impact. The color of your socks is never going to wash out your complexion.

Rule 2: The higher the color dosage, the greater the impact.

Tiny stud earrings may sit very close to your face, but even a truly dissonant color is not going to make a difference at that low of a dosage. A chunky turtleneck sweater, on the other hand, represents a much higher color dosage, so it can really make or break the look.

Taken together, the two rules of color impact have a major consequence that does not get talked about enough: There is no reason to stop wearing colors you love. Any guidelines you'll learn in this book only apply to about half of the clothes in your closet. Your pants, skirts, shoes, and accessories will not affect your color harmony.

We can also use the two rules to reduce the impact of nonideal colors. For example, if you want to wear a knit sweater in a color that is a little stark on you, you could layer a high-neck top in one of your colors underneath. That way, your neck and face don't come into direct contact with the sweater.

TRUE OR FALSE?

You can find your skin's undertone by comparing different color jewelry on your wrist or hand.

False! The first rule of color impact explains why this is a major misconception. A snippet of your skin tone, detached from the rest of your features, doesn't give you nearly enough information to infer anything about your coloring. Your face is the only true marker of color harmony.

MAX

HAIR COLOR

HEADSCARF

FOUNDATION
(UNDERTONE)

TURTLENECK

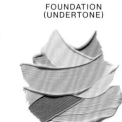

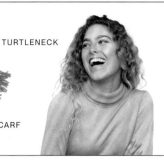

SCARF

HIGH

BACKGROUNDS (FOR
PHOTOS AND VIDEOS)

LIP COLOR
(INTENSE)

GLASSES,
SUNGLASSES

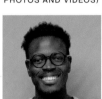

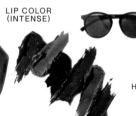

LARGE
HEADPHONES

CREWNECK TOP

HAT

MEDIUM

LARGE STATEMENT
NECKLACE

LARGE STATEMENT
EARRINGS

LOW-CUT
TOP

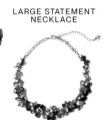

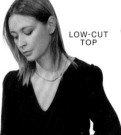

EYE MAKEUP
(INTENSE)

HAIR
ACCESSORIES

BLUSH AND
BRONZER

LOW

BRACELETS,
RINGS, WATCHES

EARRINGS
(MEDIUM)

LIP COLOR
(SUBTLE)

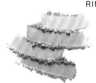

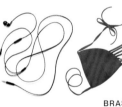

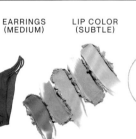

EYE MAKEUP
(SUBTLE)

HEADPHONES

BRAS, BIKINIS,
BATHING SUITS

NECKLACE

ZERO

BAGS

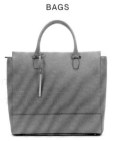

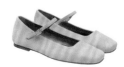

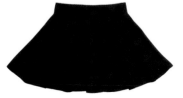

STUD EARRINGS

BODY
JEWELRY

SHOES

SKIRTS, SHORTS, PANTS

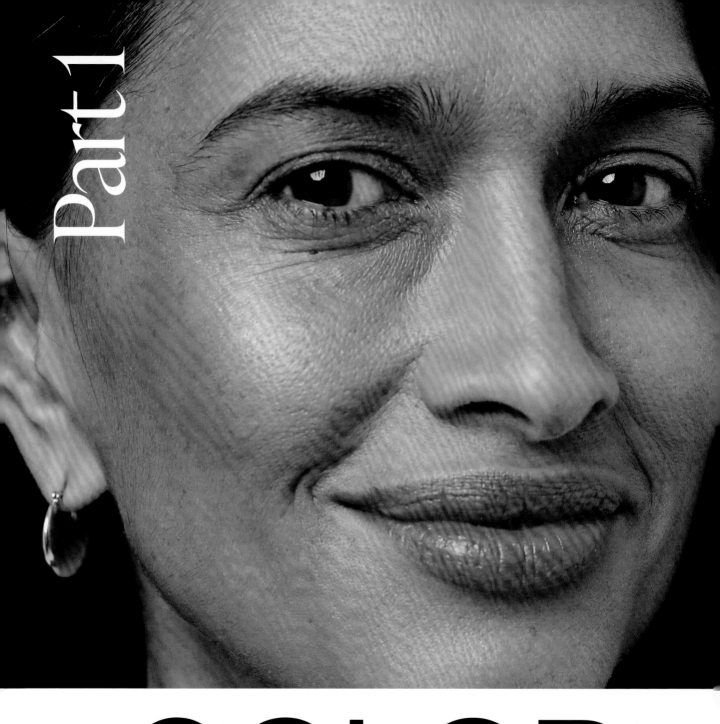

Part 1

COLOR

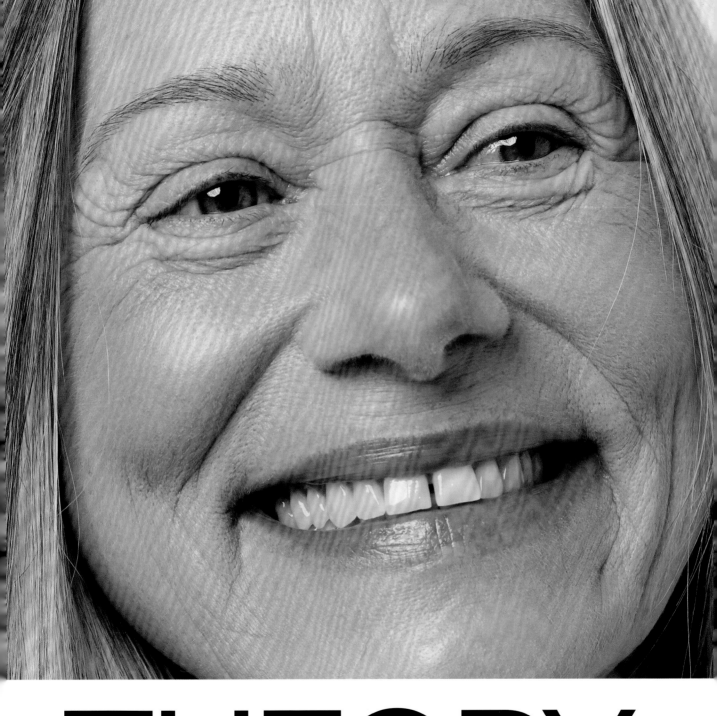

THEORY

COLOR FLUENCY

How to Read, Describe, and Differentiate Colors

How fluent are you in color? If I ask you to label this shade, are you more likely to answer "light pink with a peachy touch," or will you scratch your head and offer one or two major color groups: "It's a red-pink, maybe?"

In this chapter we will use color theory to improve your color fluency. Color fluency is about having the vocabulary and the ability to distinguish between different colors. When it comes to finding your best colors, we need to be *specific*. A "blue" sweater could look anywhere from show-stopping to jarring, depending on whether it is a robin's-egg blue, a muted periwinkle, or a supersaturated indigo. But don't worry: I won't ask you to memorize color names.

What matters is that you can "read" colors: You can look at a shade of pink and broadly situate it within the color spectrum. That you can tell whether it's more of a dusty, frosted, or vibrant pink and whether it leans more purple or red. That you can have two shades of deep green in front of you and describe what makes them different. Or that you can confidently pick out the warmest shade from a row of foundation swatches.

Color theory gives us the vocabulary we need to speak the language of colors. It provides us with a simple system for categorizing and comparing colors and everything we need to describe and assess any shade we come across.

GLOSSARY
Shade

What is the difference between a shade and a color? Strictly speaking, a shade is defined as a color that has been mixed with black. But in this book, we will keep things simple and use shade as a synonym for color.

The human eye can see about ten million different colors. But we only need three basic properties to describe and differentiate them all: hue, chroma, and value. Every color you see in the world is a unique combination of those three dimensions. And that includes the colors on your body! Just like we can use hue, chroma, and value to describe the color of the sky, the clothes in your closet, or the plants in your living room, we can use those same properties to analyze your skin tone, hair color, and eye color.

What even is color?

Before we can delve into hue, chroma, and value, let's tackle a more fundamental question: Why do things in the world even have color? The color we see is the result of light in different electromagnetic wavelengths. Red light has a different wavelength than green light, which also has a different wavelength than blue light. We can see color because our eyes have receptors (cones) that pick up these wavelengths. Light that appears white contains all wavelengths.

Think of a rainbow! Rainbows are the result of white sunlight being refracted into separate colors by tiny droplets of water in the air, which act like a prism. The rainbow rings correspond to the seven spectral colors that make up white light. The colors are always in the same order because they are arranged by wavelength. The top of a rainbow is red, which has the highest wavelength. Below red, the rainbow turns to orange, yellow, and green. Then, cyan, blue, and, finally, violet—which has the shortest wavelength—are at the bottom.

If light is the source of all color, why do things that don't emit light have a color? Everything around us, whether natural or manufactured, absorbs some wavelengths when light hits it, depending on the chemical makeup of its material. When white light (a mixture of all colors of the rainbow) hits an object, some colors get absorbed.

The receptors in our eyes pick up the wavelengths that were not absorbed, and we see the object in that color. Your T-shirt looks green because its material absorbs all wavelengths except those around 550 nanometers, which we perceive as a green color. Red paint looks red because it absorbs all wavelengths except the highest, those around 700 nanometers.

ADVANCED COLOR THEORY
Color vision can differ from person to person.

Strictly speaking, light and its different wavelengths do not have colors themselves. The specific colors we see are how our human eyes interpret these wavelengths in cooperation with our brains. Animals with other visual systems may look at the same things we do, yet see different colors. In humans, perception of color may differ due to color blindness, which affects the functionality of some or all color receptors. But even people with normal color vision may see the same color slightly differently due to variations in the shape of their retinas.

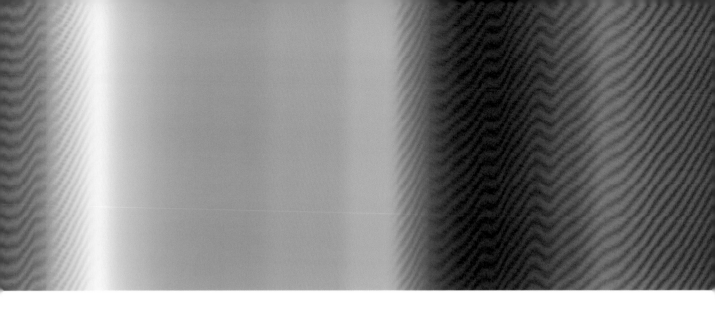

"… that sweater is not just blue, it's not turquoise, it's not lapis, it's actually cerulean."

—Miranda Priestly in *The Devil Wears Prada*

What is hue?

The hue of a color is determined by the electromagnetic waves that are picked up by the receptors in our eyes. You can think of the hue of a color as its rainbow coordinates. Rainbows are composed of seven spectral colors, but the rings of color in a rainbow are not sharp—the colors transition gently into each other, so we could divide the rainbow into infinitely more than seven colors. We could include a chartreuse and a lime between green and yellow—or a turquoise and a cerulean between the cyan and blue. The exact position a color would have among the rainbow rings is what we refer to as the hue of a color.

For the purpose of describing colors, we can group the hue spectrum into eight broad hue families:

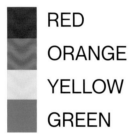 RED
ORANGE
YELLOW
GREEN

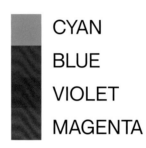 CYAN
BLUE
VIOLET
MAGENTA

Why are there eight hue families, when rainbows have seven spectral colors? You guessed it: because our hue spectrum is circular! If we could stack one rainbow on top of another, the red and violet rings would blend seamlessly, creating an eighth hue: magenta (or pink).

GLOSSARY
Grayscale shades

Black, white, and any shade of gray that can be mixed using only black and white are called grayscale shades. They are achromatic colors "without hue."

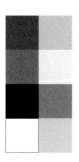

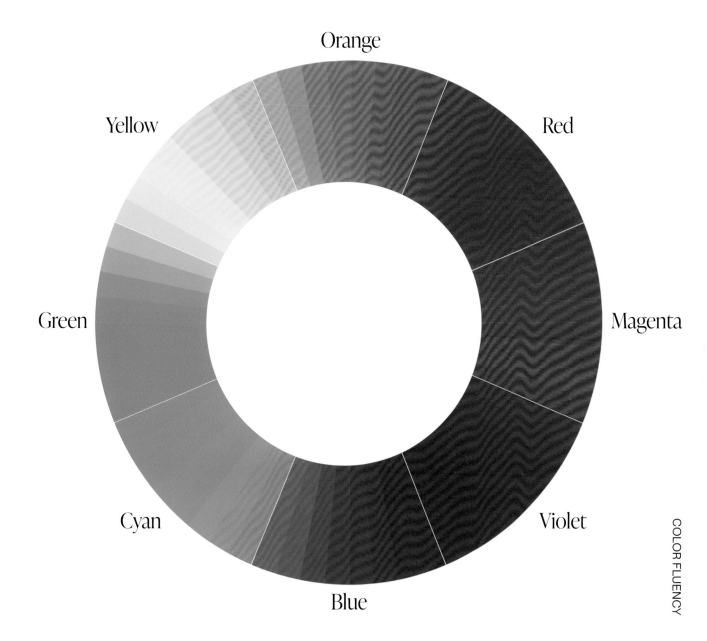

Orange

Yellow

Red

Green

Magenta

Cyan

Violet

Blue

Undertone: From cool to warm

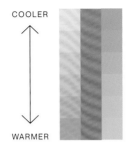

COOLER

WARMER

You already know that hue is one of the three dimensions that shape every color. But for the purpose of color analysis, we are actually more interested in a specific subcategory of hue: undertone.

All colors that have a hue also have an undertone. Undertone ranges from cool to neutral to warm, which is why it is sometimes also called a color's temperature. Like hue, chroma, and value, undertone does not exist in rigidly defined categories; it is a spectrum. In this book we will be using the following categories to describe a shade's undertone:

COOL   WARM-NEUTRAL

COOL-NEUTRAL WARM

What makes a color cool or warm?

The undertone of a shade depends on how close it is to a tangerine orange on the hue spectrum (or color wheel). You can think of that shade, right in the middle of the orange hues, as peak warmth. The further away you get from that point—in either direction of the color wheel—the cooler the shade. Both a lemon yellow and a reddish-orange are cooler than that tangerine peak. The hue on the opposite end of the color wheel is an ultramarine blue—the point of zero warmth. The closer you get to that point, the cooler the shade.

But does that mean that all blues are cool-toned and all reds are warm-toned? No! With some exceptions, all eight hue families come in cooler and warmer versions. The undertone of a specific shade depends on how it compares to other shades of the same hue family. If we say "that green has a warm undertone," we mean it is warm for being a green shade. We mean "compared to other green shades, this green is closer to the orange point of peak warmth on the color wheel." Similarly, when we refer to a "warm pink," we mean a pink closer to peak warmth than other pinks; that is, a pink that leans red instead of violet.

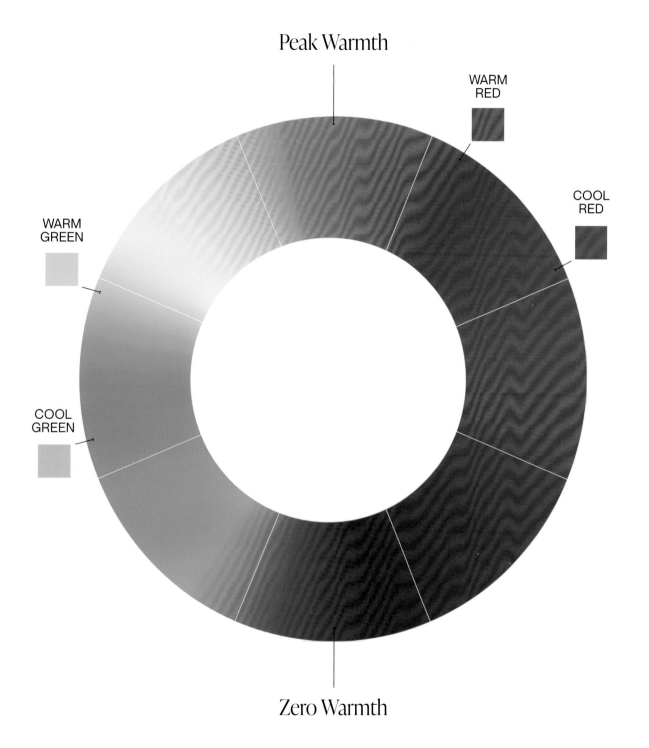

Peak Warmth

WARM
RED

COOL
RED

WARM
GREEN

COOL
GREEN

Zero Warmth

Undertone in different hues

A color's undertone depends on how close it is to peak warmth compared to other shades in its hue family. But what exactly counts as a warm red, and what as a warm-neutral red? At what point does a cool-neutral cyan become a warm-neutral cyan? In the following few pages, we'll take a look at what are typically considered cool, cool-neutral, warm-neutral, and warm versions of different hues. Keep in mind that these are guidelines only, based on my perception and interpretation of color. Someone else may categorize color slightly differently.

Red

Red hues are between orange and pink on the color wheel, so the more a red leans pink, the cooler it is. Warm reds, like tomato red, clearly lean orange. While we often think of true red as a neutral color, it actually has a slightly warm undertone. For a red color to have a cool-neutral or cool undertone, it needs to have a hint of pink in it.

LEANS PINK → COOLER
LEANS ORANGE → WARMER

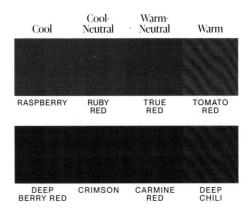

	Cool	Cool-Neutral	Warm-Neutral	Warm
	RASPBERRY	RUBY RED	TRUE RED	TOMATO RED
	DEEP BERRY RED	CRIMSON	CARMINE RED	DEEP CHILI

Orange

Since all orange hues are at the top of the color wheel cozying up to peak warmth, they can't be cool in absolute terms, and you generally won't find orange shades in the color palettes of the coolest color seasons. However, some orange shades can still be cooler than others, depending on how close they are to red or yellow.

LEANS RED OR YELLOW → COOLER

BALANCED MIX OF RED AND YELLOW → WARMER

Cool	Cool-Neutral	Warm-Neutral	Warm
	THERE ARE NO COOL OR COOL-NEUTRAL ORANGE HUES	CORAL	TANGERINE
		PAPAYA	CARROT

Yellow

Yellows are generally warm, but the more they lean into green territory, the cooler they are. A pure yellow shade (like canary yellow) that contains very little red or green is likely to be warm-neutral. Warmer yellows are halfway to orange.

LEANS GREEN → COOLER

LEANS ORANGE → WARMER

Cool	Cool-Neutral	Warm-Neutral	Warm
THERE ARE NO COOL YELLOW HUES	CITRINE	CANARY	MANGO YELLOW
	RIPE LEMON	SUNNY YELLOW	MARIGOLD YELLOW

Green

Green hues are right in the middle between peak warmth and the point of no warmth on the color wheel, so they are equally likely to be cool as warm. A green shade that looks minty has more blue, making it cooler. A chartreuse green has more yellow, making it warmer.

LEANS CYAN → COOLER

LEANS YELLOW → WARMER

Cool	Cool-Neutral	Warm-Neutral	Warm
SEAFOAM GREEN	SPRING GREEN	MANTIS GREEN	CHARTREUSE
TEAL GREEN	PARIS GREEN	FERN GREEN	LIGHT OLIVE
PERSIAN GREEN	JADE GREEN	LEAFY GREEN	KELLY GREEN

Cyan

Cyan hues are a mix of green and blue: turquoise, aqua shades, and all teals, which are simply deep cyan hues. Cyans can be cool to warm-neutral, but never warm. Cooler cyans are blues with a small amount of yellow. Warmer cyans veer toward green. Warm-neutral cyans come close to green but are still clearly distinguishable from cool-toned green hues.

LEANS BLUE → COOLER

LEANS GREEN → WARMER

Cool	Cool-Neutral	Warm-Neutral	Warm
BRIGHT SKY BLUE	BRIGHT AZURE	BRIGHT AQUA	THERE ARE NO WARM CYAN HUES
SKY BLUE	LIGHT BLUE	ROBIN'S-EGG BLUE	

Blue

The point of zero warmth is right in the middle of the blue hue spectrum. This point is an ultramarine blue that leans slightly violet and contains absolutely no yellow. Blue hues that lean violet or don't seem to contain any yellow are cool-toned. Cool-neutral blues have a hint of yellow. Any shade that contains more than a hint of yellow is likely a cyan hue. There are no blue hues that are warm-neutral or warm.

LEANS CYAN → WARMER

LESS CYAN → COOLER

Cool	Cool-Neutral	Warm-Neutral	Warm
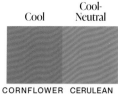		THERE ARE NO WARM-NEUTRAL OR WARM BLUE HUES	
CORNFLOWER	CERULEAN		
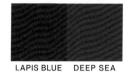			
LAPIS BLUE	DEEP SEA BLUE		

Violet

Violet hues are very close to the point of no warmth, and so more likely to be cool-toned. A less cool violet will contain considerably more red than blue: think a plum or orchid. The more blue-based a violet is, the cooler.

LEANS BLUE → COOLER

LEANS MAGENTA → WARMER

Cool	Cool-Neutral	Warm-Neutral	Warm
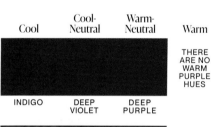			THERE ARE NO WARM PURPLE HUES
INDIGO	DEEP VIOLET	DEEP PURPLE	
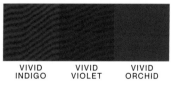			
VIVID INDIGO	VIVID VIOLET	VIVID ORCHID	

Pink

Pink (or magenta) hues are located between violet and red on the color wheel. Pinks (like greens) are halfway between peak warmth and zero warmth, meaning they are just as likely to be warm-toned as cool-toned. The closer they come to a violet, the cooler they are. Warm pinks appear reddish.

LEANS VIOLET → COOLER

LEANS RED → WARMER

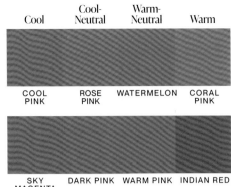

Cool	Cool-Neutral	Warm-Neutral	Warm
COOL PINK	ROSE PINK	WATERMELON	CORAL PINK
SKY MAGENTA	DARK PINK	WARM PINK	INDIAN RED

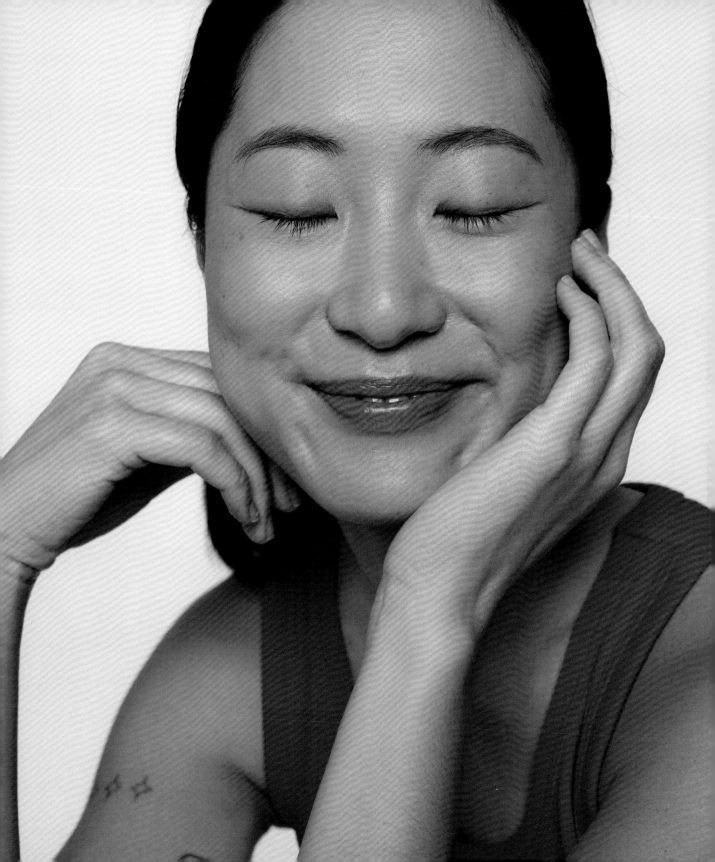

Do "neutrals" have an undertone?

Most shades we consider to be "neutrals" are very desaturated versions of one of our eight hue families. That means neutrals can be warm or cool, just like any other type of color.

Neutral Grays

Most shades of gray are not true grayscale shades—they will contain a touch of another hue, usually blue or orange. Grays that have a touch of blue (like steel, slate, or gunmetal) are cool; grays with a bit of orange will veer brown (think greige, taupe, or stone gray).

Black, white, and all true grays have a cool undertone, since they contain no amount of warmth whatsoever.

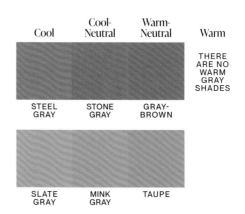

Cool	Cool-Neutral	Warm-Neutral	Warm
			THERE ARE NO WARM GRAY SHADES
STEEL GRAY	STONE GRAY	GRAY-BROWN	
SLATE GRAY	MINK GRAY	TAUPE	

Neutral Greens

When it comes to neutral greens, we have to distinguish between olive and khaki shades. Olive shades are part of the green hue family. Warm versions of these shades lean brown; cooler versions look more gray-green. A neutral green that contains more yellow than blue is likely a khaki shade. As a yellow hue, khakis are warmer the more red they contain and cooler the more green.

Cool	Cool-Neutral	Warm-Neutral	Warm
GRAY-GREEN	CACTUS GREEN	GREEN OLIVE	WARM OLIVE
THERE ARE NO COOL KHAKI SHADES	GREEN KHAKI	KHAKI	WARM KHAKI

Brown and Beige

Shades of brown generally belong to the orange hue family. The same goes for shades like cream, ivory, and beige, which are simply very light browns. Just like other orange hues, these shades are warm if they contain a balanced mix of yellow and red. If they veer more into yellow or red territory, they are cooler. Brown and beige shades are also cooler the more they lean gray (since true grays are 100 percent cool). Side note: Since the majority of browns and beiges belong to the orange hue family, the same goes for the vast range of skin tones that exist in the world. We will return to this point later on when it's time to determine the undertone of your skin.

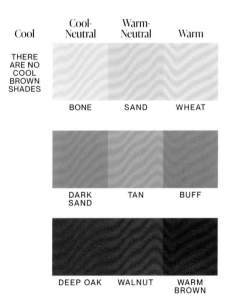

Cool	Cool-Neutral	Warm-Neutral	Warm
THERE ARE NO COOL BROWN SHADES	BONE	SAND	WHEAT
	DARK SAND	TAN	BUFF
	DEEP OAK	WALNUT	WARM BROWN

Chroma: From soft to clear

Chroma—the second of our trio of properties that determine color—tells us how colorful a shade is. Literally: How *full of color* is it? The shades we can see on a rainbow are considered *pure hues*. They show off the colors of their respective wavelengths at maximum strength. They have 100 percent chroma and are 100 percent colorful.

But the vast majority of colors we see elsewhere in the world, especially those not coming from a light or electronic source, will not be as intense and vivid. They are made up of the same hues as the rainbow rings but also contain a portion of a grayscale shade, which dilutes the color's hue and brings down its intensity.

In this book, we will be using the terms *clear* and *soft* to describe the chroma of a color. A color that is clear has high chroma and little gray. Clear colors look vivid, saturated, and intense. On the opposite end of the spectrum are soft colors, which have a higher gray percentage. Soft colors look muted, faded, and desaturated. The chroma level in between soft and clear is sometimes referred to as "neutral," but since chroma is not dichotomous (like undertone), "medium" is more accurate.

Here is a selection of colors at different levels of chroma. See if you can spot the following patterns:

☐ Clearer versions seem brighter and lighter than softer versions (although the value has been kept constant).

☐ Yellow and orange hues turn into browns and beiges at softer chroma levels.

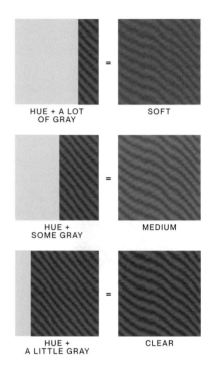

HUE + A LOT OF GRAY = SOFT

HUE + SOME GRAY = MEDIUM

HUE + A LITTLE GRAY = CLEAR

ADVANCED COLOR THEORY
Is chroma the same as saturation?

Chroma and saturation measure slightly different things, but unless you are a professional retoucher, graphic designer, or color grader, don't worry about that. Feel free to think of chroma as saturation if that makes intuitive sense to you.

Value: From deep to light

The value of a color refers to its lightness, compared to a black-to-white spectrum of achromatic (grayscale) shades. A quick way to think about the value of a color is to ask how close it is to black or white. All hues have an intrinsic value (for example, yellow shades are generally lighter than violet shades), which can be further lightened or deepened by adding white or black.

A color's chroma level can also affect how light or deep it appears: As you saw on the previous page, high-chroma (clear) shades generally seem lighter than lower-chroma (soft) shades, even when their value is the same. The most reliable way to check the true value of a shade is to remove its hue. This can be done, for example, by dialing down all saturation on an image.

The next page shows a selection of colors at different levels of value. For each, we have kept their hue and value constant. See if you can spot the following patterns:

☐ A bright yellow turns into a greenish olive shade at deeper values.

☐ Some hues appear most vivid at lighter values, while others are their clearest at deeper values (compare the yellow in the top row with the magenta in the fifth row from the bottom).

☐ Most colors appear their most saturated at medium value levels. Both very light and very deep values appear less saturated. That is because we need to add black or white to create them, which always reduces chroma.

VERY DEEP VERY LIGHT

Color genres

TEA
GREEN

PISTACHIO
GREEN

AVOCADO
GREEN

Now that you know all about chroma and value, you are ready to learn about my favorite way to understand and categorize any shade you come across: color genres. By itself, the hue of a shade tells us very little about what type of color it is. The same hue could be a pale tea green, a moderate pistachio green, and a rich avocado green—three very different shades belonging to different color "genres." If you look great in one of them, at least one of the others likely does not work that well on you. A color's genre depends on its specific combination of chroma and value. The chart on the opposite page shows the same cyan hue at three chroma levels (soft, medium, and clear) and three value levels (light, medium, and deep). We can distinguish between nine color genres:

☐ Pale Tones: light value, soft chroma

☐ Pastels: light value, medium chroma

☐ Brights: light value, clear chroma

☐ Dimmed Tones: medium value, soft chroma

☐ Moderates: medium value, medium chroma

☐ Vivids: medium value, clear chroma

☐ Dusky Shades: deep value, soft chroma

☐ Rich Shades: deep value, medium chroma

☐ Jewel Tones: deep value, clear chroma

Some of these genres will work better with your own coloring than others. For example, on my skin tone, Pastels, Brights, and Moderates look best, while Dusky and Rich Shades can be a little harsh. Most people look *great* in around two to four color genres and *good* in two to three more. If you are not sure which of the nine genres are your best, don't worry! We'll spend a good chunk of the book figuring that out. For now, let's look at some examples for each color genre so you can begin to understand them.

Chroma

	Soft	Medium	Clear

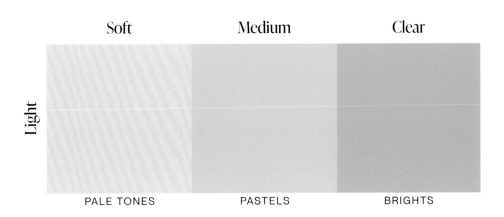

Light

| PALE TONES | PASTELS | BRIGHTS |

Value — Medium

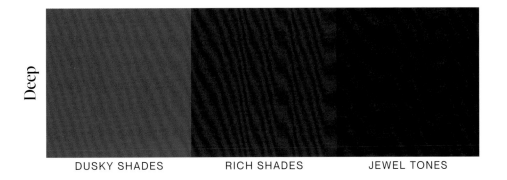

| DIMMED TONES | MODERATES | VIVIDS |

Deep

| DUSKY SHADES | RICH SHADES | JEWEL TONES |

◼◻◻ Pale Tones
◻◻◻
◻◻◻

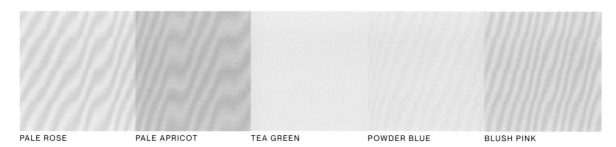

PALE ROSE   PALE APRICOT   TEA GREEN   POWDER BLUE   BLUSH PINK

Any light shade with a hint of hue is a Pale Tone, from icy pale pinks to faded heather grays. All light grays and light neutrals belong to this color genre, including the light tan shade of classic trench coats and chinos. All almost-whites—like off-white, ecru, and vanilla—are Pale Tones. Pale Tones are sometimes mislabeled as "Pastels," which are more saturated and encompass their own color genre.

◻◼◻ Pastels
◻◻◻
◻◻◻

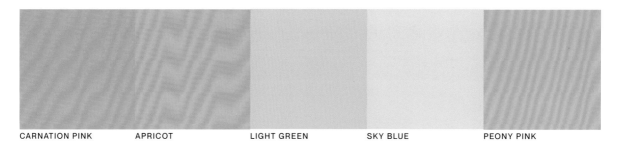

CARNATION PINK   APRICOT   LIGHT GREEN   SKY BLUE   PEONY PINK

Pastels have a light value and a medium chroma, like the crisp green of a Granny Smith apple. If a shade is light, contains no visible amount of gray, and does not appear close to max saturation, it's likely a Pastel. The majority of Pastels are too saturated to be considered neutral, except for some more saturated beige shades.

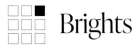

Brights

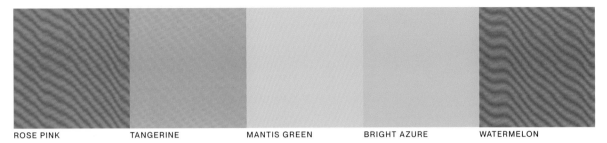

ROSE PINK   TANGERINE   MANTIS GREEN   BRIGHT AZURE   WATERMELON

Brights—light shades with a clear chroma—are strictly non-neutral. Many of the most vibrant items you'll find in clothing stores are Brights, as are most vibrant yellow and orange shades, since these hues appear to be most saturated at lighter values. I also consider pure white a (cool-toned) Bright, due to its total lack of gray.

Dimmed Tones

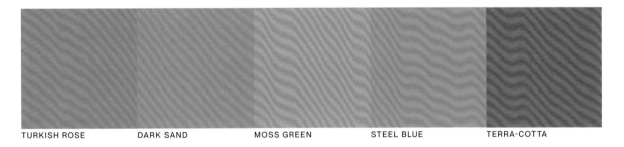

TURKISH ROSE   DARK SAND   MOSS GREEN   STEEL BLUE   TERRA-COTTA

Dimmed Tones have a medium value and a soft chroma—think stone-wash medium denim. Many shades that are considered neutrals are a part of this color genre: all medium-value grays, many lighter browns, khakis, olives, and muted blues. Dimmed Tones are often described as muted, diffused, subdued, or faded.

▣ Moderates

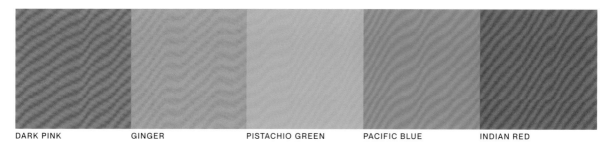

DARK PINK   GINGER   PISTACHIO GREEN   PACIFIC BLUE   INDIAN RED

Moderates have both a medium value and chroma. Despite what the name may suggest, they are still one of the more "colorful" genres and don't include many neutrals. Warm green, yellow, and orange Moderates will appear somewhat more muted since these hues peak in saturation at higher values. Due to their mid-range value and chroma, Moderates are one of the two color genres (along with Rich Shades) that come closest to being universally flattering.

▣ Vivids

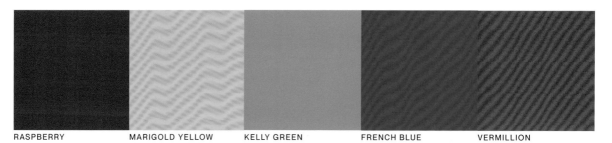

RASPBERRY   MARIGOLD YELLOW   KELLY GREEN   FRENCH BLUE   VERMILLION

Since most colors show off the full magnificence of their hues at medium values, Vivids are statement colors by design. Vivids contain minimal gray, white, or black; they come closest to the pure hues of the rainbow. Any color that can be described using the terms vibrant, bold, ultra, shocking, brilliant, electric, or hot may be a Vivid shade. Note: This does not include neon and fluorescent colors. Ultrabright shades like these are not found in nature, so while they can look fine on some people, they aren't fully harmonious on anyone.

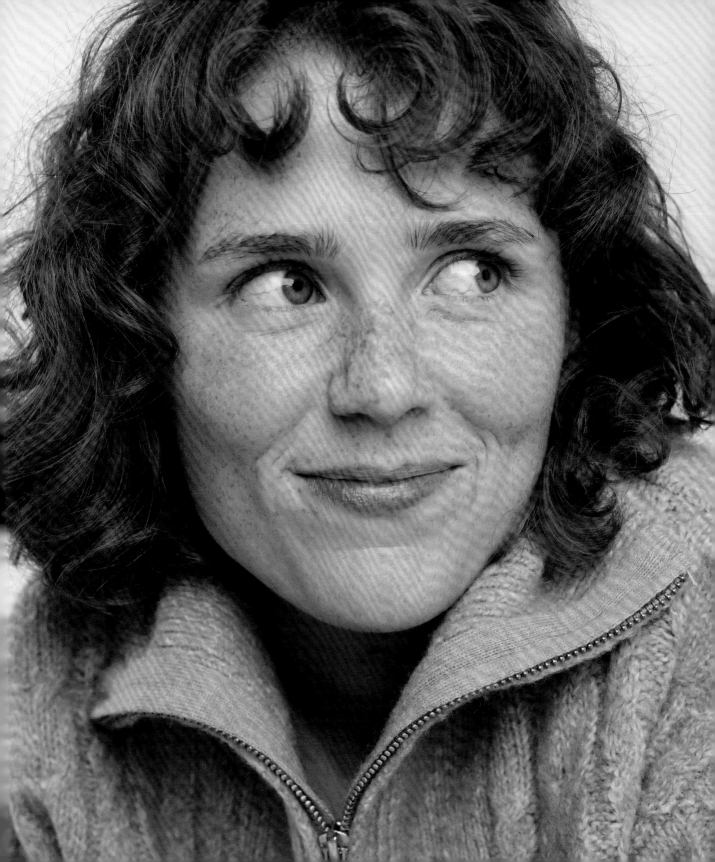

Dusky Shades

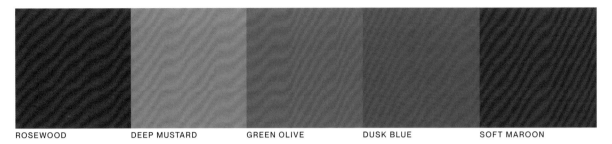

ROSEWOOD   DEEP MUSTARD   GREEN OLIVE   DUSK BLUE   SOFT MAROON

Dusky Shades have a deep value and a soft chroma. They may also be described as smoky, burned, or muddy. Any shade that has a deep gray base with just a touch of hue is likely a Dusky Shade. This includes many browns, neutral greens, and deeper grays. In clothing, Dusky Shades tend to be top-sellers since they feel inconspicuous and distinctly non-flashy. Paradoxically, since colors like dusk blue, gray-brown, and deep mustard exist on the outer edge of the value/chroma spectrum, they are far from universally flattering.

Rich Shades

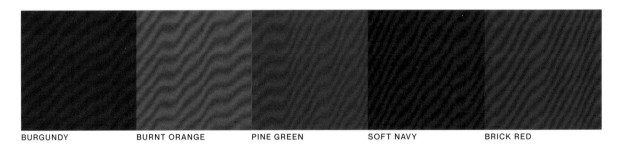

BURGUNDY   BURNT ORANGE   PINE GREEN   SOFT NAVY   BRICK RED

Like Moderates, Rich Shades are neither particularly vivid nor subdued. Any deep color that is neither gray-adjacent nor vibrant is likely a Rich Shade. This also includes most almost-black shades like dark eggplant, as very deep shades have limited saturation, even when they don't contain gray. For the same reason, pure black is a (cool-toned) Rich Shade.

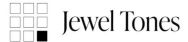 Jewel Tones

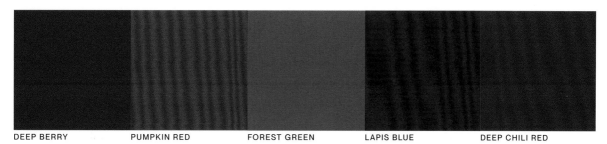

DEEP BERRY   PUMPKIN RED   FOREST GREEN   LAPIS BLUE   DEEP CHILI RED

Jewel Tones are maximally saturated at a deep value. Like gemstones, they carry maximum intensity, but if you compare them to Vivids, you'll see that they appear a little less colorful. Yellow hues do not exist in this genre, since they appear brown at lower values.

COLOR HARMONY

Why You Can Predict Which Colors Will Work on You

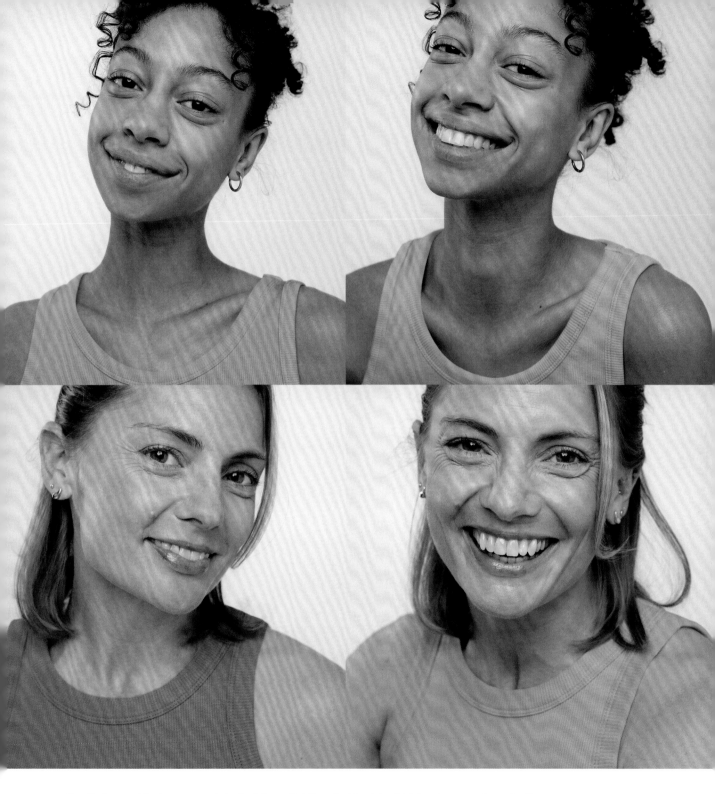

Camille (top row) looks gorgeous in both pictures. But if you had to pick, which top do you prefer on her? Intuitively, which color do you think works better on Caroline (bottom row)?

That some colors look good on you and some don't is not random. There is a pattern. Color harmony is the secret to finding colors that light you up, instead of wash you out. It's the reason your friend looks fresh and glowy in the same pastel-hued duffle coat that just doesn't suit you. But what exactly is it about the color of that duffle coat that makes it look harmonious on your friend but not on you? And how can you predict how well a shade is going to work on you without trying it on? That's what we'll cover in this chapter.

But before we can figure out why certain colors look better on some people than others, we need to answer another question first: What makes certain color combinations work better than others?

Let's do a little experiment! On the right, you can see three color palettes in two versions. Which versions do you prefer?

Color harmony would predict you picked version A for each palette because they are more cohesive. Cohesion is what makes it look like a harmonious theme of shades rather than a random, mismatched mix. What do the terms *cohesive, harmonious,* and *matching* all boil down to? Similarity. A cohesive color combination is one where the shades are all similar in some way.

As we have already learned, a color can be similar to or different from another based on three aspects:

1   UNDERTONE: How cool vs. warm is this color?

2   CHROMA: How soft vs. clear is this color?

3   VALUE: How light vs. deep is this color?

Colors harmonize when they echo each other in undertone, chroma, or value—when they are all similarly cool or warm, deep or light, or clear or soft. Colors clash or look dissonant when none of their properties align, when there is no common thread that connects them.

Let's take another look at our sample palettes and look for that common thread. In the first palette, the shades are all soft and medium-value, with a neutral to warm undertone. The vivid, cool pink in version B sticks out like a sore thumb. That same pink feels right at home in the second palette, where all shades are similarly clear and cool.

In the second palette, swapping out the rich peacock blue on the right for a paler glacier blue does not look bad per se, but it does break the theme. That same glacier blue feels much more at home in the third palette, consisting of cool, muted, mid-range shades. If we swap the blue for the dark peach of the first palette, it looks off.

A   B

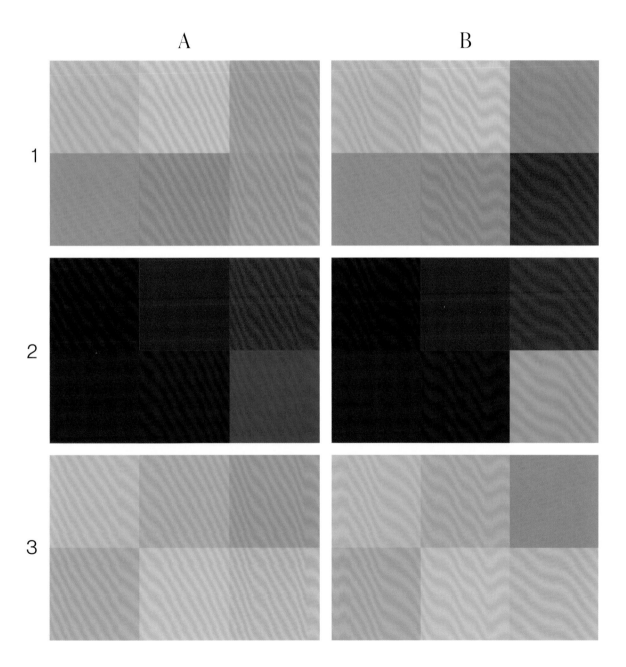

1

2

3

Why do we find cohesive color schemes harmonious?

The rich, dusky hues of a sunset, the dimmed, golden tones of autumn leaves on a forest floor, or the hazy grays and blues of a misty lake: nature is full of harmonious color schemes. Our brains respond to color harmony the same way they respond to symmetry, balance, contrast, and several other principles that have been found to be pleasing to the human eye across cultures and throughout history.

The jury is still out on exactly why we like cohesive color schemes. Our preference for color harmony could have evolved as a way to avoid potentially unsafe environments or foods. Or it could be related to our brain's massive reliance on pattern recognition. We make sense of the world by spotting patterns and discrepancies in those patterns. Our brains may have developed a preference for anything that our visual system can identify as a pattern by rewarding us with a pleasurable feeling. That could be why seeing a harmonious color scheme feels satisfying—like all the puzzle pieces fitting together.

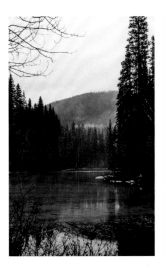
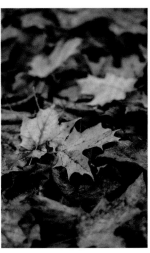
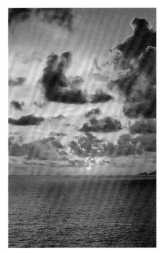

Don't complementary colors go well together?

Colors that sit opposite each other on the color wheel are considered complementary colors. Fashion, art, and interior design experts tend to recommend pairing complementary colors, such as blue and orange, because they often look great next to each other. But doesn't that recommendation go against everything we have discussed so far? How do complementary colors—shades from the opposite ends of the color wheel—fit in with the concept of color harmony, which states that similar colors go well with each other?

The answer is that the two concepts pertain to different aspects of color. Whether two shades are complementary depends on their hue: for example, any green hue is complementary to any pink hue. But whether two shades are *cohesive* depends on their undertone, chroma, or value. For example, carnation pink harmonizes with an equally cool and bright seafoam green, but less so with a dusky warm olive. Many notable works of art are a wild mix of hues from all around the color wheel: think of Van Gogh's *The Starry Night*. It is colorful and contains several complementary colors. But it still looks harmonious because there is a common thread among the specific shades.

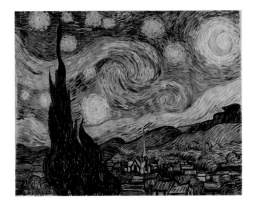

Why some colors look better on you than others

Whenever we are wearing a color, whether in the form of a sweater, an eyeshadow, or a hair color, we are adding that color onto the canvas of our own face and body. And that canvas already contains an established color scheme: Your skin tone, eye color, and natural hair color are all perfectly harmonious, and will fall somewhere on the spectrum of cool to warm, soft to clear, and deep to light.

Colors that echo and honor your own natural coloring with respect to their undertone, chroma, and value will look harmonious and effortless on you. Colors that go against your natural coloring will feel less intuitively satisfying. They will stick out, like the "wrong" color in the B versions of our sample palettes on page 51.

For example, if your skin tone, eye color, and hair color have an obvious cool undertone, you will shine in shades that are similarly cool. Warm colors, on the other hand, may clash a little with your skin tone. Or, if your coloring is soft and muted, similarly gentle shades will complement you the most, while brighter, more vivid colors may overwhelm you.

Let's examine how this works in real life. Anja has warm-toned blond hair, light aqua eyes, and a porcelain skin tone. Her light eyes and hair create a low contrast against her fair skin. Overall, her coloring has a warm-neutral undertone, a medium chroma, and a light value.

Anja looks gorgeous in both pictures, but the cool, deep purple top in the left-hand picture overwhelms her delicate complexion. The pistachio-colored top, on the other hand, creates a beautifully cohesive combination with her fair, delicate coloring. Just like her natural coloring, Anja's best colors have a warm-neutral undertone, a medium chroma, and a light value.

Her most dissonant colors have the opposite of her coloring's properties: cool, very clear or very soft, and deep.

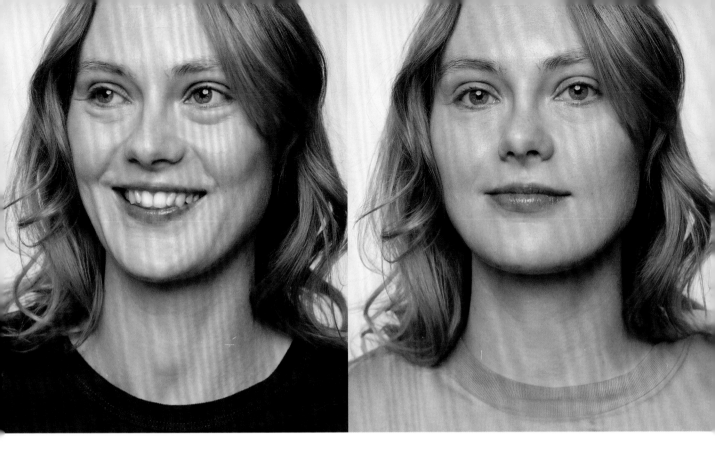

	Anja's coloring	Harmonious colors	Dissonant colors
UNDERTONE	warm-neutral	warm-neutral	cool
CHROMA	medium	medium	very soft or very clear
VALUE	light	light	deep

Best

Opposite

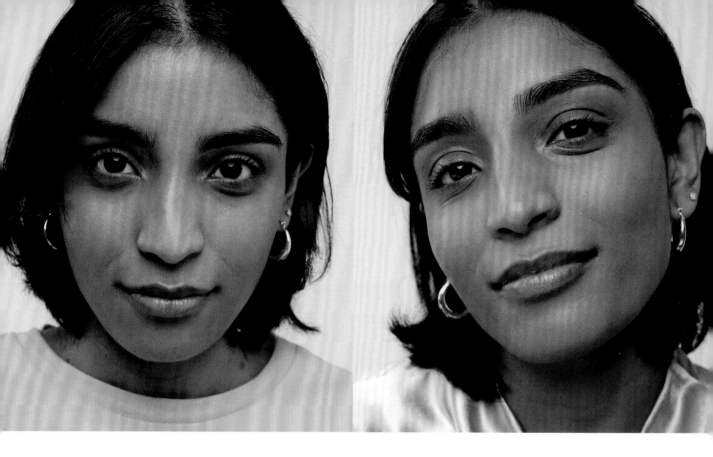

	Kripa's coloring	Harmonious colors	Dissonant colors
UNDERTONE	cool	cool	warm
CHROMA	clear	clear	soft
VALUE	medium-deep	all values	—

Best

Opposite

You shine in colors that echo and honor your unique color essence.

Kripa's rich black hair and black-brown eyes create a high contrast with her cool, medium skin tone. Her overall coloring is cool, clear, and medium-deep. Compare these two colors on Kripa: a cool silver on the right, and a pale apricot on the left. Both photos were taken in the same light and Kripa looks stunning in both of them. But the cool, bright silver works better with her clear, cool coloring, while the pale apricot can't really keep up with her. Kripa's best colors have a cool undertone and a clear chroma—just like her coloring. Her most dissonant colors have the opposite of her coloring's properties: warm and soft.

Why the value of your best colors depends on your contrast level

"But wait a minute," you might be thinking. "Aren't silver and pale apricot both light colors? Why does one work and the other doesn't? And isn't Kripa's coloring on the deeper side, which should harmonize better with deeper colors?" Good catch!

Determining the undertone and chroma of your best colors couldn't be more straightforward: If your coloring is warm and soft, your best colors will be as well. But it doesn't work the same way with value. This is because most of us are not all light or all deep—our coloring contains various values. Plus, not everyone with a deep coloring is suited to only deep colors, and not everyone with light coloring is suited to only light colors. In fact, quite often, the people who look great in the absolute deepest shades (like black) also look amazing in the absolute lightest (like white). What type of people can pull off intensely contrasting colors? Those who already possess a lot of contrast naturally. On the other side of the spectrum are the people with a more blended coloring who do best with shades that don't create much contrast against their skin.

The more contrast you possess naturally, the greater the range of values you can pull off.

Anja's best colors are light, not because her coloring is light overall (although it is). It is because her contrast level is low, which means she is suited to colors that do not create much of a value contrast against her skin tone.

And what about Kripa? Her contrast level is high, which is one reason she looks great in all values, from the deepest to the lightest. Other factors also play a role, and we will discuss these later. But for now, all you need to remember is that we will not be trying to determine an overarching value for your coloring. Instead, we will look at your contrast level to find your ideal value range: How deep are the deepest shades and how light are the lightest shades that harmonize with your coloring?

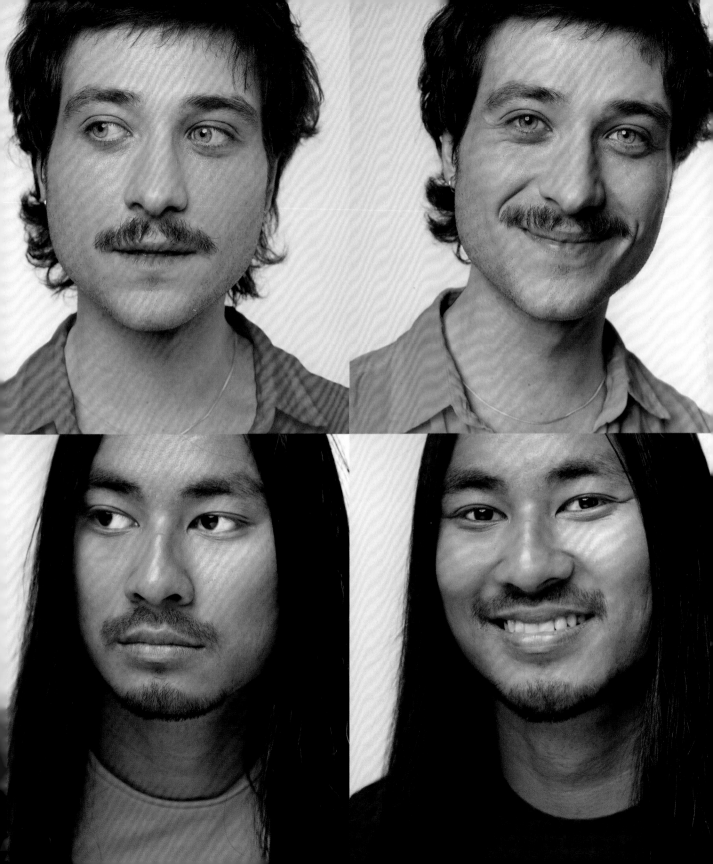

COLOR TYPES

What the Twelve Seasons Have to Do With Color Theory

When color analysis first hit the scene, it was an in-house service. An image consultant would come to your home, sit you down in front of a mirror, and proceed to drape you in a variety of colored fabrics to demonstrate which colors flattered you and which didn't. Based on the results, they'd assign you a season, like Winter, and hand you a small set of color swatches that you could take shopping with you. You'd know your type, you'd know your colors, and you just hoped that image consultant knew what they were talking about.

Fast-forward a few years. As mentioned, Carole Jackson released a book, *Color Me Beautiful,* that became an instant bestseller. Now, you no longer had to hire an image consultant—you could figure out your color season by yourself and then just skip to the relevant chapter to find all your best colors. Readers were still not told why these colors supposedly suited their season. But *you* know why, because now you know all about color harmony: Readers were recommended color palettes that echoed their own coloring in terms of undertone, chroma, and value/contrast. The twelve different seasons in color analysis all correspond to a specific combination of those three dimensions. For example, a True Winter corresponds to a cool undertone, clear chroma, and high contrast level. A Light Spring corresponds to a warm-neutral undertone, medium chroma, and low or medium contrast level. This chapter is designed to give you a broad overview of this system of seasons and address a few common misconceptions before you start figuring out your own season in Part 2.

The four original seasons

The original typology outlined in *Color Me Beautiful* consisted of only four seasons: Spring, Summer, Autumn, and Winter. Instead of contrast, value was used as the third variable determining one's season and was mostly based on hair color.

	Spring	Summer	Autumn	Winter
UNDERTONE	warm	cool	warm	cool
CHROMA	clear	soft	soft	clear
VALUE	light	light	deep	deep

Depending on their season, people were recommended one of four color palettes. The Spring color palette consisted of warm, clear, and light shades, such as coral, peach, turquoise, pastel yellows, and light greens. The Summer palette featured softer, muted shades with cool undertones—think soft blues, lavenders, lighter grays, and dusty pinks. Someone who was assigned the Autumn season was recommended rich, earthy colors like deep oranges, rusty reds, olive greens, and golden browns. The Winter palette was the boldest and most dramatic of the palettes, with high-contrast shades like white, black, jewel tones, and vivid pinks and purples.

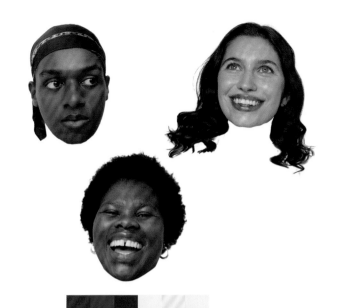

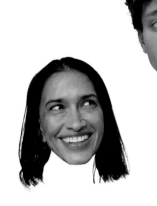

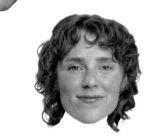

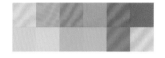

Winter

COOL CLEAR DEEP

Spring

WARM CLEAR LIGHT

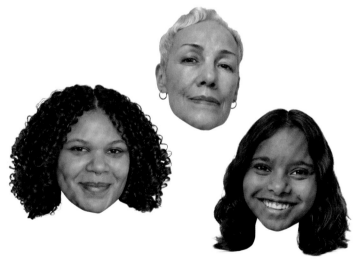

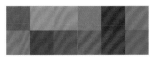

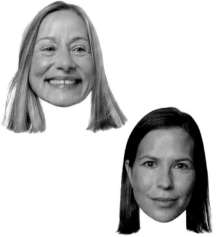

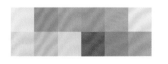

Autumn

WARM SOFT DEEP

Summer

COOL SOFT LIGHT

From four to twelve seasons

Since the 1980s, each of the four original seasons has been refined into three seasons.

☐ The Spring season has been divided into Clear Spring, True Spring, and Light Spring.

☐ The Summer season has been divided into Light Summer, True Summer, and Soft Summer.

☐ The Autumn season has been divided into Soft Autumn, True Autumn, and Deep Autumn.

☐ The Winter season has been divided into Deep Winter, True Winter, and Clear Winter.

Expanding the system to twelve seasons ultimately leads to more people getting better color recommendations. The twelve-season typology accounts for the fact that not all Winters, for example, will be equally cool, clear, and deep. Since all three variables exist on a spectrum, some people's coloring will fall in the middle of a season, while others lean more toward one side. For example, a Winter type that is deep but less clear will be suited to different colors than one that is very clear but less deep. The new typology distinguishes between these types, such as Deep Winter and Clear Winter, and offers a more fine-tuned color palette for each.

In the four-season model all color dimensions were treated as binary: you were either cool or warm, soft or clear, and deep or light. The new system allows for more nuance and acknowledges that some people's undertone, chroma, or contrast level may well be "somewhere in the middle."

Clear Winter

COOL-NEUTRAL
CLEAR
HIGH/MEDIUM

Clear Spring

WARM-NEUTRAL
CLEAR
HIGH/MEDIUM

True Winter

COOL
CLEAR
VERY HIGH/HIGH

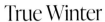

True Spring

WARM
CLEAR
MEDIUM/LOW

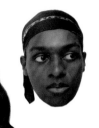
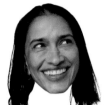
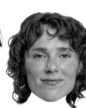

Deep Winter

COOL-NEUTRAL
MEDIUM
VERY HIGH/HIGH

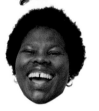

Light Spring

WARM-NEUTRAL
MEDIUM
MEDIUM/LOW

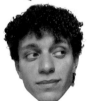

Deep Autumn

WARM-NEUTRAL
MEDIUM
VERY HIGH/HIGH

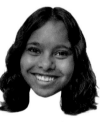

Light Summer

COOL-NEUTRAL
MEDIUM
MEDIUM/LOW

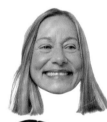

True Autumn

WARM
SOFT
VERY HIGH/HIGH

True Summer

COOL
SOFT
MEDIUM/LOW

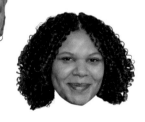
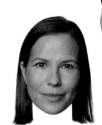

Soft Autumn

WARM-NEUTRAL
SOFT
HIGH/MEDIUM

Soft Summer

COOL-NEUTRAL
SOFT
HIGH/MEDIUM

Why are the prefixes of the seasons not consistent?

Why is there a Soft Summer, but no Soft Winter or Soft Spring? The prefixes of the twelve new seasons are based on an older, now outdated concept: dominant traits. The theory was that every person's coloring would be pronounced in one of six ways: warmth, coolness, clarity, softness, depth, or lightness. That dominant trait would then determine their season. For example, a Light Spring's coloring was thought to be characterized by the light value of their skin, hair, or eyes. Since Spring types are always warm, clear, and light, there cannot be a Soft Spring, Cool Spring, or Deep Spring.

Most color analysts no longer consider the dominant trait theory to be accurate or helpful. Light Springs are not always especially light; their coloring is simply in between that of a True Spring and a Light Summer. Also note that, in this book, we are not using the overall value of someone's coloring to determine their season at all. Instead, our third color dimension is contrast (see opposite for more). You do not need to have a light overall value to be one of the two Light seasons (Light Spring or Light Summer). Almost any skin tone can be a Light season if their contrast level is low or medium. The same goes for the two Deep seasons; they are characterized by a very high or high contrast level, not a deep overall value.

Color dimensions of each season

In color analysis, you'll often see the color seasons arranged in the form of a circle because that is a helpful way to illustrate how the seasons relate to and flow into each other. A season's position within that circle (or matrix) tells us everything we need to know about its three color dimensions: undertone, chroma, and contrast. Let's take a closer look at each.

Undertone

Undertone is represented by two diagonal axes connecting the four True types: True Spring, True Summer, True Autumn, and True Winter. The four True types are the only seasons that have an obviously cool or warm undertone. All other types are only slightly cool or slightly warm.

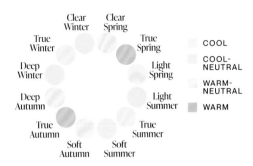

Chroma

The y-axis of the circle illustrates the seasons' chroma: The four seasons at the top have a high (clear) chroma, while the four seasons at the bottom have a low (soft) chroma. The two Deep and the two Light seasons in the middle of the chart have medium chroma.

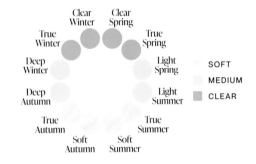

Contrast

Unlike undertone and chroma, a season's contrast level consists of a range. Two people can share a season, but have different contrast levels. In this book, we will distinguish between four contrast levels from very high to low. Each season corresponds to two contrast levels, represented by the x-axis of the circle: The four seasons on the left (True Autumn to True Winter) have the highest contrast level: either very high or high. The four seasons on the far right (True Spring to True Summer) are medium or low contrast seasons. The middle group (Clear Winter and Clear Spring, and Soft Summer and Soft Autumn) are either high or medium contrast.

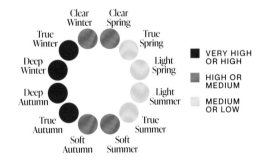

Does every season have a specific "look"?

Considering how specific each season's dimensions are, you may assume that people who belong to the same season are going to look pretty similar. But nothing could be further from the truth. People can have very different features, yet belong to the same season and be suited to the same colors. The models opposite have different skin tones, different eye colors, and different hair colors. And yet they are all suited to the same palette of cool, brilliant shades of True Winter. With one exception, any skin tone can be any season.* Any eye color and most hair colors can be any season. While some seasons have a narrower range than others, there is diversity in every season.

Sister seasons

Seasons that sit next to each other on the seasonal matrix are called sister seasons, and they share enough similarities to be able to borrow from each other's color palettes. For example, the sister seasons of True Spring are Clear Spring and Light Spring.

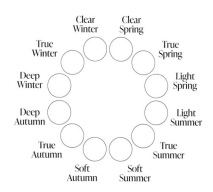

The closer seasons are on the seasonal matrix, the more they have in common and the more their color palettes overlap. For example, you can see that the Deep Winter type is closer to the Deep Autumn than to Clear Winter. For this reason it is important that we don't think of the twelve seasons as "sub-seasons" of one of the original four seasons, but as stand-alone color types. The Deep Winter and Deep Autumn seasons have just as much in common as Deep Winter and True Winter do (or any other neighboring seasons). Because each of the twelve seasons are separate types, don't attempt to determine your "main season" first and then pick a sub-season.

---

* People with a rich-deep skin tone are unlikely to be one of the low/medium contrast seasons, since their skin tone will usually create at least a high contrast against their teeth and the whites of their eyes.

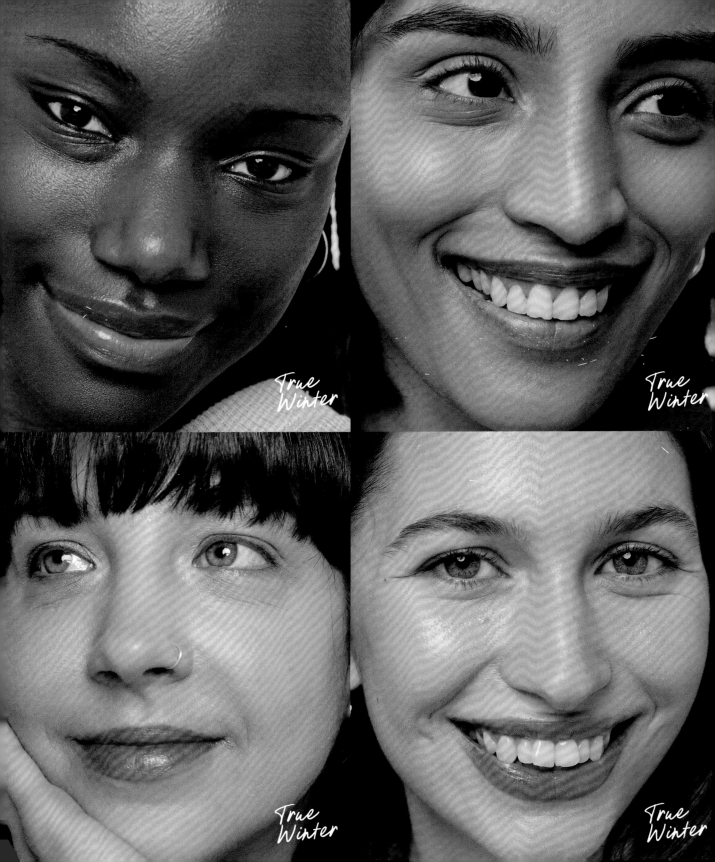

True Winter

True Winter

True Winter

True Winter

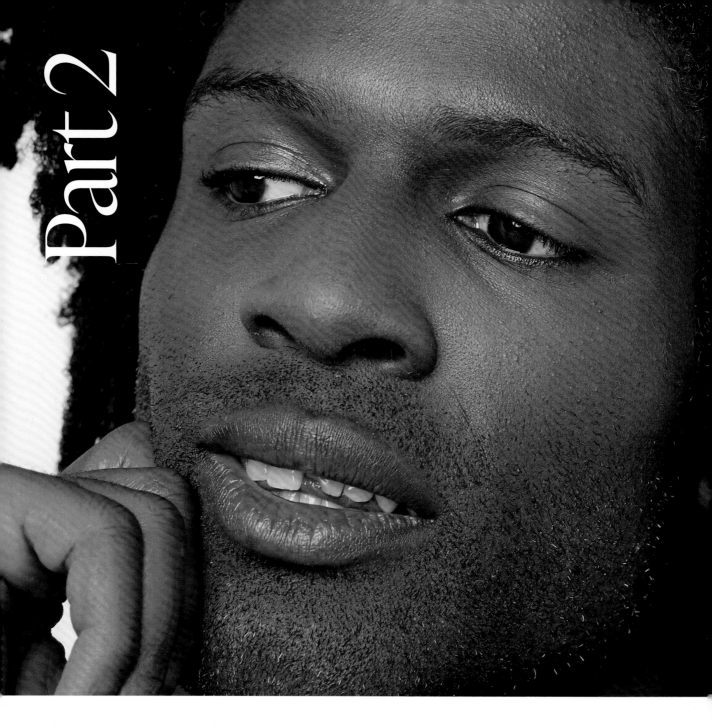

Part 2

FIND YOUR

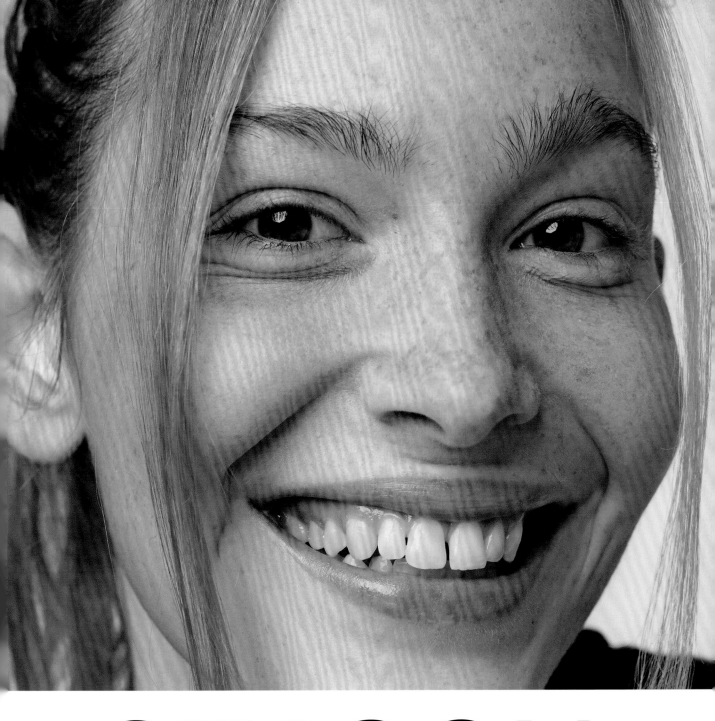

SEASON

ROAD MAP

How to Find Your
Season in Five Steps

Do you know your contrast level? Is your undertone cool, warm, or somewhere in between? Is your chroma soft or clear? Now that you've mastered color theory, you're well on your way to answer all of those questions confidently and accurately. In this chapter we'll take a bird's-eye view at the five steps it takes to determine your color season. We'll go into more detail for each step in the sections and chapters that follow. Are you a True Spring? A Soft Summer? Let's find out!

Step 1: Take photos of your coloring

Finding your season is like solving a case: You need to collect evidence, analyze that evidence, and then put all your findings together to arrive at the solution. Your evidence is your coloring, and your investigation depends on you being able to see your coloring clearly and accurately. Bad lighting and even subtle color casts can botch the entire case.

For best results, I recommend you take photos of your coloring and use them instead of the mirror to assess your contrast, undertone, and chroma in the next steps. That way, you'll only have to worry about lighting once, and you can use your phone to check whether your photos have any sort of color cast. Later in this chapter, you'll learn exactly how to take your pictures and ensure they accurately capture your coloring.

Step 2: Find your contrast level

Start the investigation by assessing your contrast level. Is it very high, high, medium, or low? Your goal is to exclude at least two of these categories. To determine your contrast level, you need to assess the value of your skin tone and then compare it to the value of your hair and eye color. To a lesser degree, you will also take into account your eyelashes and eyebrows.

CATEGORIES: Very high, high, medium, or low

RELEVANT FEATURES: Skin tone, hair color, eye color, eyebrows and eyelashes

Step 3: Determine your undertone

Next, you'll analyze whether your undertone is cool, cool-neutral, warm-neutral, or warm. While it's great if you can pinpoint your undertone exactly, narrowing it down to two out of the four categories is enough at this stage. Your skin tone will be the key factor here and your natural hair color may provide bonus evidence. Your eye color is not a good indicator of your undertone (more on this later).

CATEGORIES: Cool, cool-neutral, warm-neutral, or warm

RELEVANT FEATURES: Skin tone and hair color

Step 4: Figure out your chroma

The last attribute—your chroma—tends to be the hardest for most people to determine. We'll use your skin tone and eye color to estimate your chroma: Is it soft, medium, or clear? Your goal is to exclude at least one of these categories. Your hair color sits this one out.

CATEGORIES: Soft, medium, or clear

RELEVANT FEATURES: Skin tone and eye color

To grasp the power of color harmony, you need to see it with your own eyes.

Step 5: Test out colors to confirm your season

Once you have completed your preliminary investigation, you will be able to narrow down your list of potential seasons to three to six final contenders. But analyzing your coloring can get you only so far. To crown your winning season—and feel confident about your choice—you need to try on different colors and examine how they work on you in the flesh. Even if you think you know how certain colors look on you, to grasp the power of color harmony, you need to see it with your own eyes. That's where draping comes in: In the world of color analysis, draping refers to the practice of holding a piece of fabric to your face to test how well it harmonizes with your coloring. Professional color analysts usually have ready-made fabric strips (drapes), but any item that's made from fabric can serve as a drape. In a pinch, you can even use non-fabric objects to test a specific color. In a later chapter, you'll learn all about how to hold your very own at-home draping session, which colors to test out, and how to interpret the results to determine your season.

How your age impacts your coloring

Your skin tone, eye color, and hair color change throughout your life. Let's discuss what this means for your color analysis.

If you are under the age of fifteen, or if you are a parent or relative trying to type a child, please be aware that your or your child's coloring may change quite dramatically with age. A child's coloring has very little relevance to their color season as an adult. You may have been blond as a five-year-old, but that does not make your adult-age dark brown strands any less high-contrast.

Past puberty, your coloring (specifically your chroma and contrast level) will continue to change—though rarely enough to alter your color season. In other words, if you are a True Spring at twenty, you will still be a True Spring at seventy, regardless of whether you dye your hair, eyebrows, or eyelashes. Your very best colors will likely shift a little, though (we will discuss this in detail in later chapters). Regardless of age, if you determine your color season based on what you see in the mirror right now, you can't go wrong.

How to capture your coloring on camera

The very first step of your color analysis is to take a few photos of your skin tone, hair, and eye color. You can take all of your pics by yourself and in one go, using the camera on your cellphone. But remember: These photos are not just regular old selfies—they are evidence! They form the basis of every step that follows, so it's crucial that they represent your coloring clearly and accurately. Let's talk about exactly what you'll need to capture.

How many photos do I need to take?

I recommend you take four photos:

☐ One of your whole face

☐ One of your side profile

☐ A close-up photo of your eye region

☐ A photo of the top of your head, allowing you to see your hair close up

Where should I take my photos?

Outside in natural daylight under a clear sky, or indoors facing a window. Avoid sunrise, sundown, the "golden hour," direct sunlight, or an overcast day. Make sure your face is well lit but not in bright, direct sunlight. There should be no warm, glowy hue on your face from the sun.

Can I take the photos myself?

You can use the camera on your cellphone to take your pics or get someone else to take them for you. Either way, make sure your shots are close-ups: Your face should cover more than two-thirds of the frame, and your eyes should be in focus. Someone who doesn't know you should be able to tell your eye color from looking at each of your pics.

Where should I face in relation to the light?

You want your face to be evenly lit from the front, so turn your whole body toward the sun or window, then hold up your camera to take your pics. The light should not come from behind you.

☐ In natural daylight, your coloring is captured accurately.

☐ On an overcast day, your photo may turn out too dark with a grayish blue tint.

☐ Direct sunlight acts like a warm filter over your coloring.

☐ Indoor lighting may give your coloring a yellow to blue tint.

What should I wear?

Your photos should ideally contain no colors other than those of your skin, hair, and facial features, so wear a low-cut top that won't show up or can be cropped out. Take off all jewelry, glasses, and makeup.

Does it matter how I pose?

Whether you smile or not is up to you. What matters is that both your irises and the whites of your eyes are clearly visible. Depending on your eye shape, you may need to pretend you just saw something truly shocking for your pics.

Is there anything else I need to pay attention to?

Yes! Make sure you've turned off your phone's flash and any blurring or "beautifying" filters.

Is it okay if I wear a little makeup?

No, sorry! It's important that you capture your coloring at its factory setting. That means absolutely no makeup. No tinted lip balm or CC cream or dab of concealer allowed—even if you think it matches your skin tone perfectly.

If you have any form of permanent makeup on your face (including microbladed eyebrows), you will have to base your analysis on what you looked like without it. I recommend you find multiple older pictures of yourself to keep on hand during the analysis. If your lashes or eyebrows are tinted, I recommend you take your pictures when the tint has faded completely.

To find your season you need to capture your coloring at its factory setting.

Can I wear self-tanner?

Absolutely not! Even a small amount of self-tanner can alter your skin tone considerably. If you regularly use self-tanner of any kind, make sure there are absolutely no traces left when you take your pictures.

What about a natural tan?

If your skin tans in the sun, I recommend you analyze your coloring when you have as little of a natural tan as possible. Although a natural tan does not alter your undertone as much as a self-tanner, it still makes it considerably more challenging to assess your natural undertone and chroma accurately.

What if my hair is color-treated?

Your natural hair color is an essential criterion for assessing two out of the three dimensions (undertone and contrast). If your hair is color-treated (even minimally), you will still need to base your analysis on your original hair color. Even subtle babylights can affect the accuracy of your analysis, as any type of lightening warms up the hair.

But don't just *assume* what your hair color looked like before coloring—get hard, photographic evidence. Perhaps you also have a close relative who shares your hair genes? If so, find a photo of their hair color to use throughout the next steps.

What about gray or white hair?

Although hair that has fully transitioned to gray or white will harmonize with the rest of your coloring, I generally recommend people base their analysis on the natural hair color they had before going gray. If your hair color is evidence, hair that has gone gray is a bit like an evidence report with a ton of redacted information. It doesn't point us in the wrong direction, necessarily, but it also doesn't give us much to work with. For example, gray hair does not allow us to infer anything about value and contrast level, and it's also usually not a great indicator of undertone because of its super-low chroma.

It is absolutely possible to determine someone's season based on gray or white hair without knowing their prior hair color, but it is harder because part of the evidence has been redacted.

How should I wear my hair for the pics?

If your hair is not color-treated it is a key piece of evidence, so leave it down.

If your hair is color-treated or gray, please do not cover it up with a towel or other piece of fabric (which would add another random color into the mix). Instead, put it up in a tight bun or slick it back with some gel.

Your turn

Here are your to-dos for this chapter:

☐ Plan out where and when you are going to take your photos.

☐ Make sure you have no traces of self-tanner or makeup on your face when you take your photos.

☐ Take four close-up photos:

A photo of your whole face

A photo of your side profile

A photo of your eye region

A photo of the top of your head, allowing you to see your hair close up

☐ Check your photos to make sure they accurately reflect your coloring.

☐ If applicable, collect multiple older photos of your natural hair color and/or your face without permanent makeup. Keep in mind that analogue photos can fade or develop a yellow tint over time.

YOUR CONTRAST LEVEL

Very High, High, Medium, or Low?

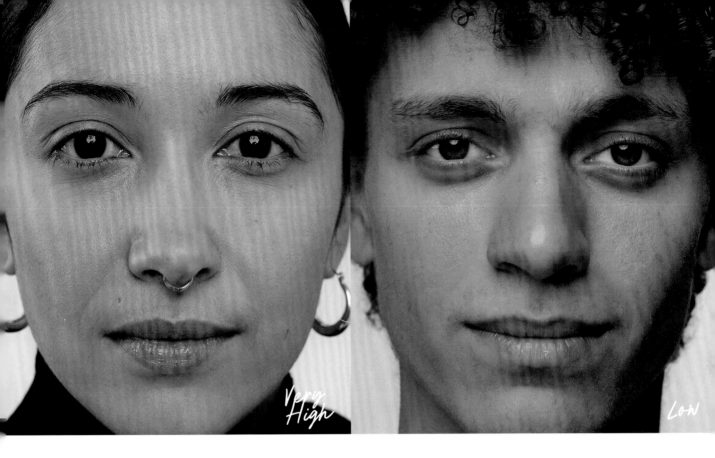

Very High

Low

Compare Jess (left) and Amin (right). Both have a light-medium skin tone, but the rest of their features are very different. Jess's hair and eye color create a strong contrast against her skin, and her eyebrows and lashes give her even more definition. Amin's hair and eyes are not much deeper than his skin.

CATEGORIES: Very high, high, medium, or low

RELEVANT FEATURES: Skin tone, hair color, eye color, eyebrows and eyelashes

Your contrast level depends on the amount of contrast your hair, eyes, and other features create against your skin tone. Contrast is a measure of intensity. If your contrast level is high, your coloring naturally possesses a lot of definition and depth; if your contrast level is low, your coloring is more delicate and blended. Contrast is independent of skin tone: With some exceptions, all skin tones can have any contrast level.

Contrast is closely related to *value,* which signifies how deep or light a color is, from black to white. All colors fall somewhere on that scale, including the color of your skin, hair, and eyes. Your contrast level depends on the difference in value between your skin tone and the rest of your features, mainly your hair and eye color, but also your eyebrows, eyelashes, teeth, and the whites of your eyes. The greater the difference, the higher your contrast level.

To figure out your contrast level, you need three pieces of information:

☐ How deep is your skin tone, from rich-deep to fair?

☐ How deep is your natural hair color, on the hair level scale of 1 to 10?

☐ What is your exact eye color: black-brown, brown, hazel, green, blue, or gray?

In the first half of this chapter, you'll determine each of these one by one. Your skin tone, hair level, and exact eye color are all key features that you will keep referring back to throughout the book, so take your time and make sure you feel confident about your assessment before moving on. In the second half of this chapter, you will use all of the information you gathered to calculate your contrast level.

Your contrast level has a big influence on the range of values that harmonize with your coloring. The greater your contrast level, the greater the range. If you naturally possess a lot of contrast, you'll look great in colors that are quite a bit deeper or lighter than your skin tone. On the other hand, if your coloring is low-contrast, you'll do best with shades that are not much lighter or deeper than your skin tone.

Your contrast level is also a good indicator of how much intensity you can pull off when it comes to makeup. People who naturally possess a lot of contrast can handle intense definition, deep shades, and bold lip colors, while lower-contrast folk often feel like even subtle makeup looks harsh on them.

Your skin tone

In this book, we will use seven categories to describe skin-tone depth:

RICH-DEEP	LIGHT-MEDIUM
DEEP	LIGHT
MEDIUM-DEEP	FAIR
MEDIUM	

Take a look at the models on the next page representing each category. Although their features and complexions vary, you can see how their skin tone has a similar depth. Now compare those images to the photos you took of your own coloring. Which category best matches your own skin tone, in terms of its value (deep to light) only? Ignore all other features and color dimensions (such as contrast, chroma, or undertone). If your skin tans in the sun, pick the category that matches your skin when it does not have a tan.

Go by the images only, not the category names! Brands and beauty professionals all use different systems to classify skin tones, so just because your foundation is labeled "light-medium" does not mean your skin will fall into the Light-Medium category in this book.

Skin tones

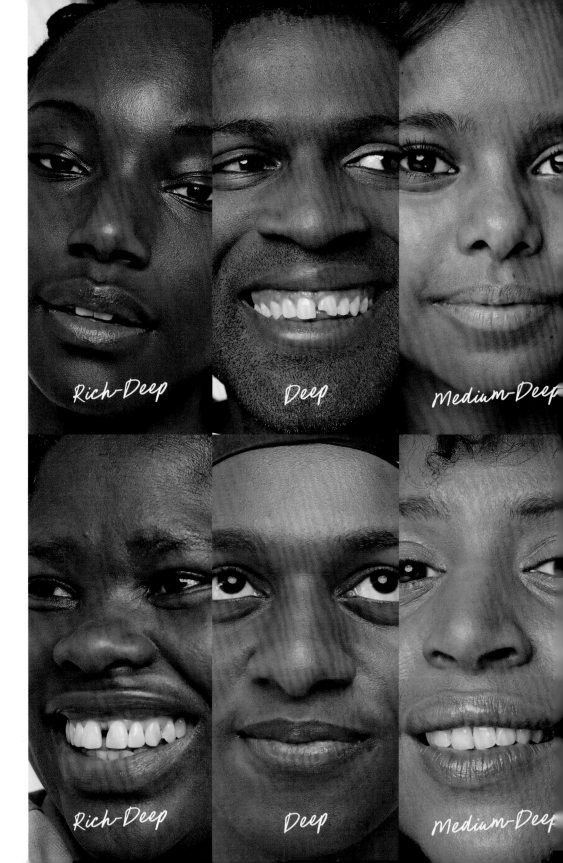

Rich-Deep

Deep

Medium-Deep

Rich-Deep

Deep

Medium-Deep

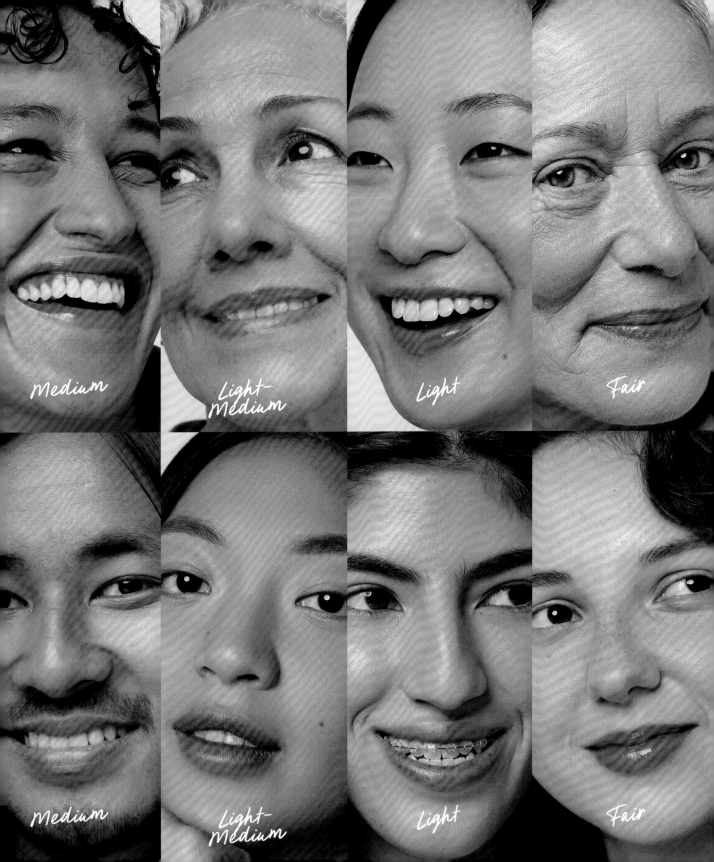

Medium

Light-Medium

Light

Fair

Medium

Light-Medium

Light

Fair

Your hair level

To classify the value of your natural hair color, we will borrow a concept that is used by hairstylists and colorists throughout the world: hair levels. All hair colors from black to the lightest blond can be assigned a level from 1 to 10. Hair level depends solely on the value of the hair, regardless of its tone or hue; for example, a bright copper shade and an ashy dark blond are both a hair level 7.

To determine your hair level, compare the photos you gathered of your natural hair color (as an adult) to the swatches on the opposite page. Remember, we are only focusing on how light or deep the hair is, regardless of undertone, chroma, or hue. Focus on the hair near your crown! Ignore any bits that seem lightened from the sun, the ends, and any finer hairs around your hairline.

Unless you are a hair professional, make sure you go by the pictures, not the names of the hair levels! You may find that what you have been calling "medium brown" hair is considered a "dark blond" in the world of hair professionals. If you have red hair of any kind, be careful that you are not overestimating your hair level, because the high saturation of your hair can make it seem quite a bit brighter than its actual value.

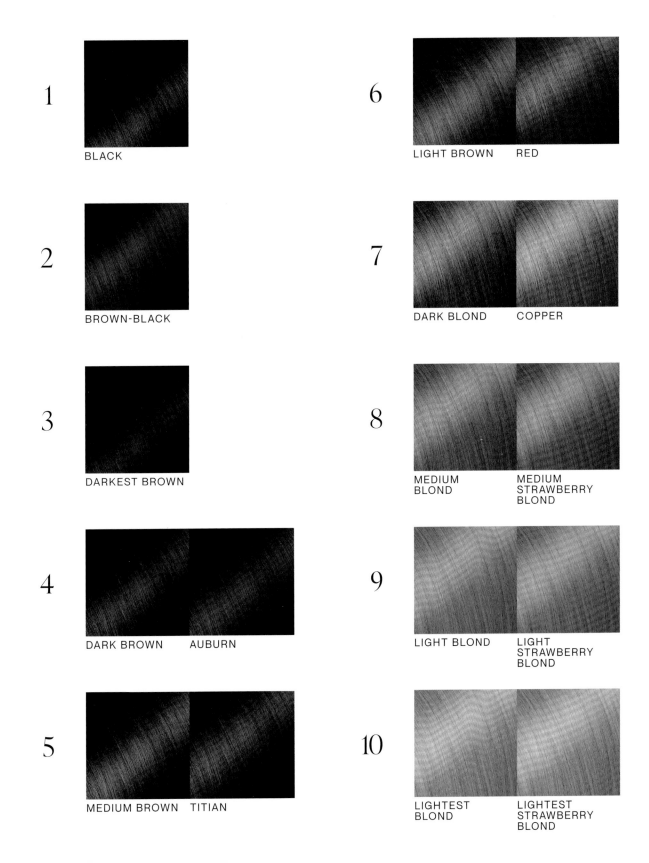

1 BLACK

2 BROWN-BLACK

3 DARKEST BROWN

4 DARK BROWN AUBURN

5 MEDIUM BROWN TITIAN

6 LIGHT BROWN RED

7 DARK BLOND COPPER

8 MEDIUM BLOND MEDIUM STRAWBERRY BLOND

9 LIGHT BLOND LIGHT STRAWBERRY BLOND

10 LIGHTEST BLOND LIGHTEST STRAWBERRY BLOND

Your eye color

Throughout the book, we will use six general eye colors: black-brown, brown, hazel, green, blue, and gray. Do you know which of these best represents your own eye color? If not, compare the close-up picture you took of your eyes to the images below to find your closest match.

☐ BLACK-BROWN: Your brown eyes are very deep, with hardly any hints of red or yellow.

☐ BROWN: Your eyes are a light, medium, or deep brown that does not fit the black-brown or hazel eye criteria.

☐ HAZEL: Your eyes are a light brown shade that leans green.

☐ GREEN: You have light to deep green eyes with no hints of brown or blue.

☐ BLUE: You have light eyes with a subtle to strong blue hue. If your eyes look blue-green, pick this category.

☐ GRAY: If your eyes are light but you can barely spot hints of blue and see no green, you have gray eyes!

When in doubt…

Here's what to pick when you can't decide between two or more shades.

BLACK-BROWN OR BROWN → BROWN

BROWN OR HAZEL → BROWN

HAZEL OR GREEN → HAZEL

GREEN, BLUE, OR GRAY → BLUE

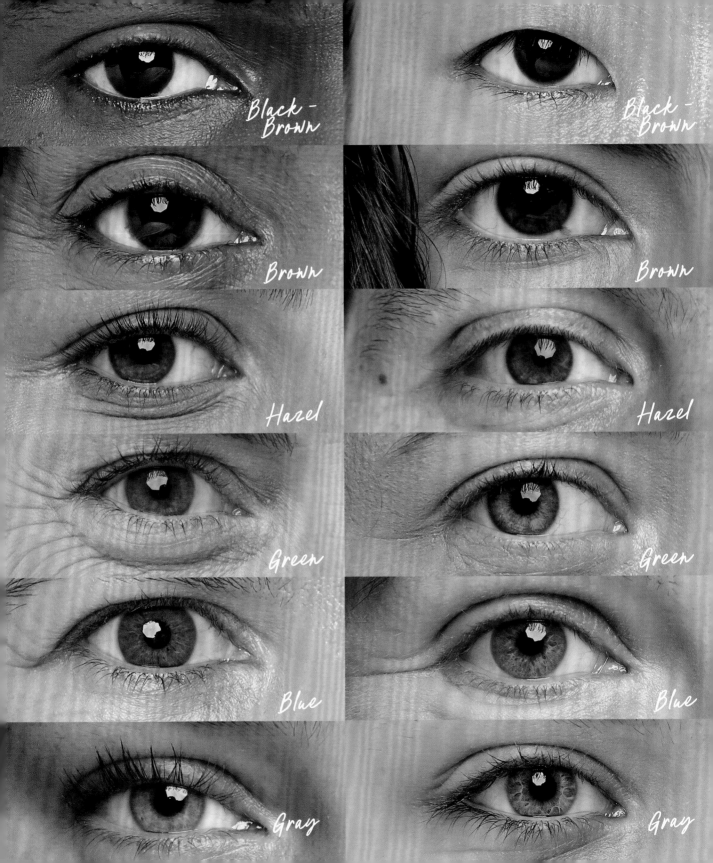

Black–Brown

Black–Brown

Brown

Brown

Hazel

Hazel

Green

Green

Blue

Blue

Gray

Gray

What determines your eye color?

Your eye color is largely determined by the concentration of the pigment eumelanin on the front and back of your iris. Since eumelanin is brown or black, the more your eyes contain, the deeper they will be.

Blue, green, and hazel eyes are also a consequence of eumelanin, or rather a lack thereof. Our eyes do not contain blue or green pigment. There is either eumelanin or there is none. When eyes have no or very little eumelanin in the front of the iris (the stroma), they will look blue because of a light effect called Rayleigh scattering, which is also responsible for the sky looking blue. When eyes contain a small amount of eumelanin, that bit of brown gets mixed with the blue and your eyes appear green. Hazel eyes are the result of a moderate amount of eumelanin.

Green eyes that have a stronger golden tinge, as well as some brown eyes, do contain another pigment—lipochrome—which has a yellow hue. Gray eyes are thought to differ from blue eyes by the amount of collagen in the stroma, resulting in the light being scattered slightly differently.

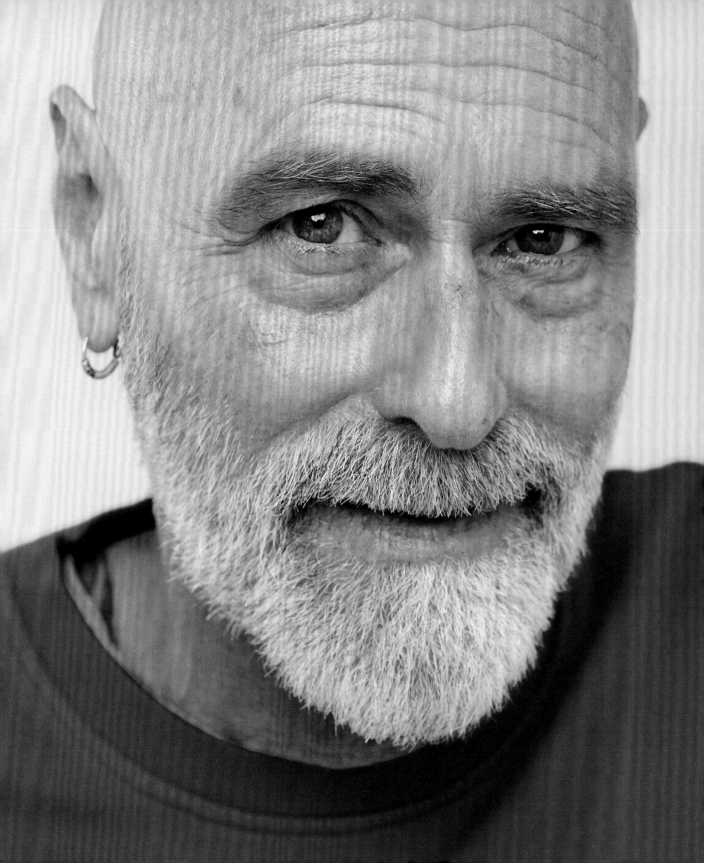

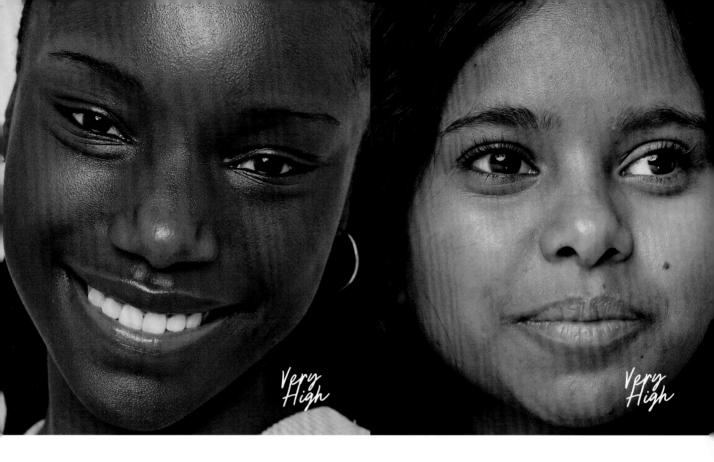

Very High

Very High

Contrast in rich-deep, deep, and medium-deep skin tones

If you have a rich-deep, deep, or medium-deep skin tone, you can exclude certain contrast levels right off the bat. If your skin tone is rich-deep, your contrast level is either high or very high. If your skin tone is deep or medium-deep, its contrast is either very high, high, or medium, but never low—regardless of your hair color or other features. This is because deeper skin tones will always create a certain level of contrast against the whites of your eyes and your teeth.

Is your contrast level very high?

If your contrast level is very high, both of the following must be true:

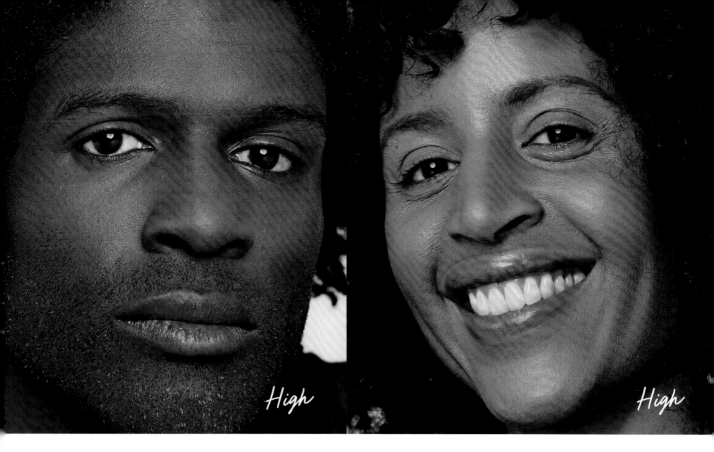

High

High

☐ Your eyes are black or black-brown (not brown).

☐ Your eyebrows and eyelashes add a lot of extra contrast and intensity to your face.

If either of these is not true and your skin tone is rich-deep, your contrast level is high, not very high.

Is your contrast level medium?

If your skin tone is deep or medium-deep, your contrast level could be medium if both of the following are true:

☐ Your hair is lighter than a level 2 (not black or black-brown).

☐ Your eyes are light (not black-brown or brown).

If either one of these is not true, your contrast level is high.

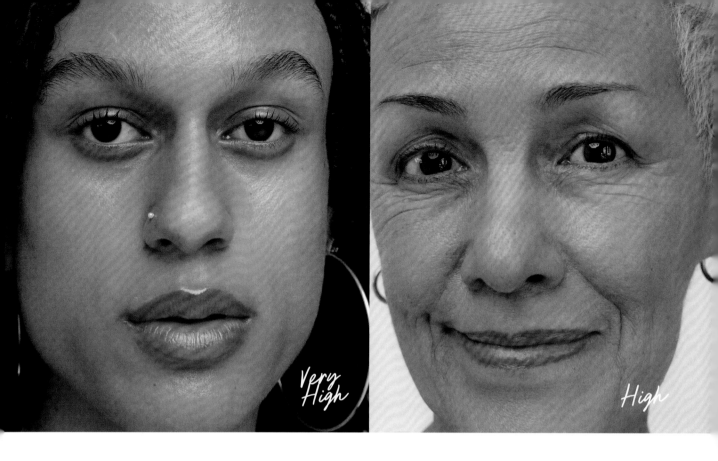

Very High

High

Contrast in medium and light-medium skin tones

For medium skin tones—medium or light-medium—a high contrast is most common, followed by very high contrast. Medium contrast is less common, and low contrast levels are rare.

Is your contrast level low?

Your contrast is low if all of the following are true:

☐ Your eyes are light (not black-brown or brown).

☐ Your hair is a level 6 or above (light brown or lighter).

☐ Your eyebrows and eyelashes are not very prominent.

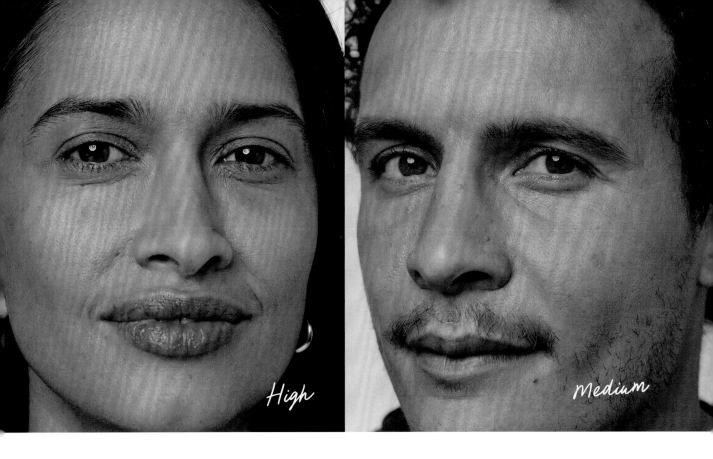

High   *Medium*

Is your contrast level medium?

Your contrast level is medium if all of the following are true:

☐ Your eyes are light (not black-brown or brown).

☐ Your hair is a level 3 or lighter (darkest brown or lighter).

Is your contrast level very high?

Your contrast level may be very high if the following are true:

☐ Your hair is a level 1 or 2 (black or black-brown).

☐ Your eyes are black-brown.

If neither is true, your contrast level is high.

Contrast in light and fair skin tones

People with light or fair skin tones can have any contrast level from very high to low. However, high and medium contrast levels are considerably more common than very high and low contrast levels.

Use the table below to check how much contrast your hair level creates against your skin tone. Regardless of your eye area, your contrast level is at least that. For example, if you have level 6 hair and light skin, your contrast level is at least medium. If your hair is a level 4 and your skin is fair, your contrast is at least high. However, your overall contrast could also be one level higher than that if your eye area adds a lot of definition to your face.

Hair level	Light	Fair
1	very high	very high
2	very high	very high
3	high	very high
4	high	high
5	medium	high
6	medium	medium
7	low	medium
8	low	low
9	low	low
10	low	low

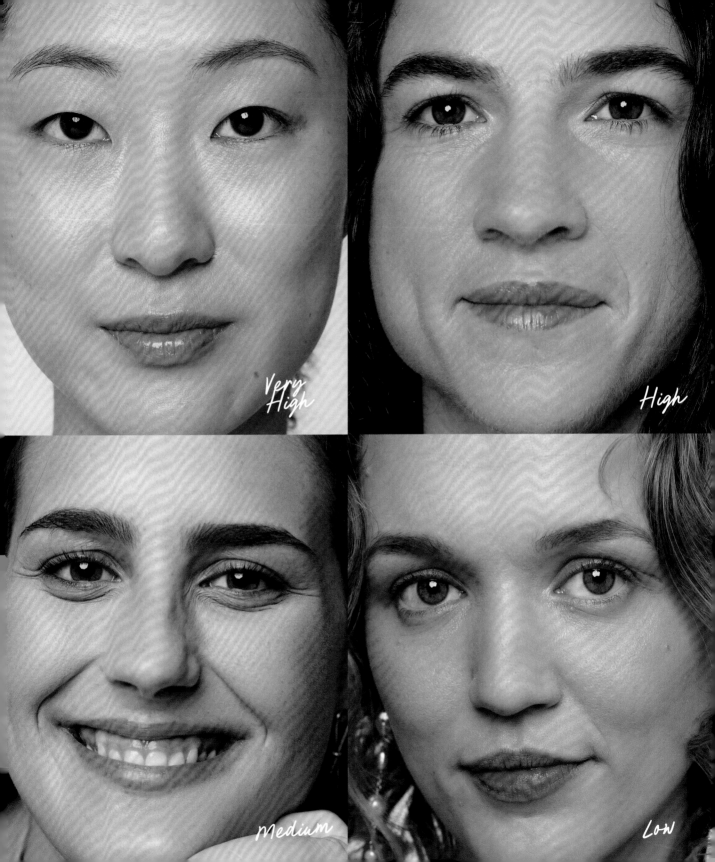

Very High

High

Medium

Low

Is your contrast level high or very high?

If your hair creates high contrast against your skin, your overall contrast level is very high if any of the following are true:

☐ Your eyes are black-brown.

☐ Your eyes are brown, and your eyebrows and eyelashes are very prominent.

Is your contrast level medium or high?

If your hair creates medium contrast against your skin, your overall contrast level is high if:

☐ Your eyes are brown or black-brown.

Is your contrast level low or medium?

Low contrast levels are quite rare, even in light and fair skin tones. Even if your hair creates low contrast against your skin, your overall contrast level is medium if any of the following are true:

☐ Your eyes are a deep version of brown, hazel, green, blue, or gray.

☐ There is an obvious dark ring around your iris.

☐ Your eyebrows are naturally prominent and quite a bit darker than your hair color.

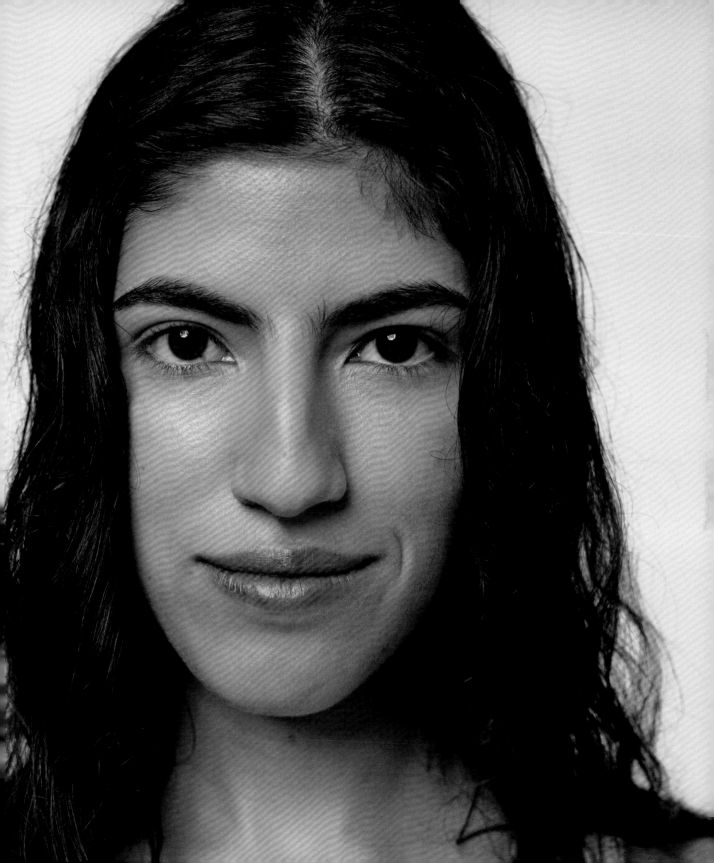

YOUR UNDERTONE

Cool, Cool-Neutral,
Warm-Neutral, or Warm?

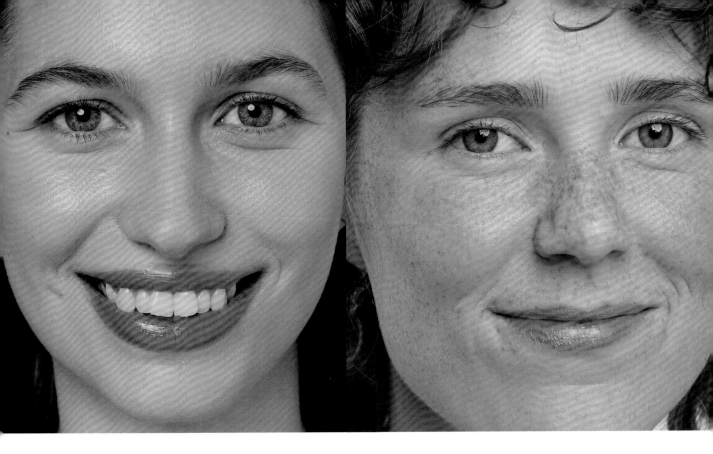

Tordis (left) and Lena (right) are on opposite ends of the undertone spectrum. Although Lena's skin is fair, it is obviously warm. Her copper hair is the definition of warmth. Compare that to Tordis: Her hair is a cool medium-brown, her skin an alabaster shade. Note also how Lena and Tordis both have blue eyes. Contrary to popular belief, blue eyes are common among people of all undertones and are not an indicator of a cool undertone.

CATEGORIES: Cool, cool-neutral, warm-neutral, or warm

RELEVANT FEATURES: Skin tone and hair color

Your undertone depends on the amount of warmth in your skin tone and natural hair color. If you can spot of a lot of orange warmth, your undertone is warm; if you can barely detect any hints of warmth, your undertone is cool. Most people fall somewhere in the middle and have either a cool-neutral or a warm-neutral undertone. In line with color harmony, the undertone of your coloring is also the undertone of your best colors. For example, if your coloring is warm, you will shine in the warm versions of any hue. If your coloring is cool-neutral, you'll shine in the cool-neutral shades, and so on.

Undertone is undoubtedly the celebrity among the color attributes: Not only does it get the most attention, it's also the one with the most rumors about it. Perhaps you've heard through the grapevine that "the color of your veins can help you find your undertone" or "if you tan easily, you are warm" or "fair skin is usually cool and deeper skin is usually warm." None of those rumors are true!

For the record: Almost all skin tones are just as likely to be warm-toned as cool-toned (with the exception of rich-deep skin tones, which are slightly less likely to have a warm undertone). Whether you burn or tan or do neither in the sun also has nothing to do with your undertone, just the amount of pigmentation in your skin. And the color of your veins is the result of so many different factors, from the value of your skin to its chroma, that you really can't use it to infer anything about your undertone.

But don't worry, even without these little shortcuts, finding your undertone can be quite straightforward—once you know what to look for. In this chapter, we'll dive into how undertone shows up in skin and hair—and what exactly counts as cool, cool-neutral, warm-neutral, and warm. Your eye color does not reflect your coloring's overall undertone, so will not factor in (more on this on page 106).

Your goal for this chapter is to home in on two of the four undertone categories. For example, if you end up feeling certain you are either cool-neutral or warm-neutral, that is all you need at this stage. Or if you know you are definitely not warm but can't quite decide between cool-neutral or cool: perfect! You'll figure out the rest later on.

Undertone in skin

Whether your skin has a cool or warm undertone comes down to a single factor: warmth. To understand what that warmth looks like, we need to familiarize ourselves a little with the biology of our biggest organ. The color of your skin largely depends on the amount and ratio of two types of pigments—eumelanin and pheomelanin—that are produced by specialized cells in the bottom layer of the epidermis. Of course, many other factors, from hormones to UV exposure to medication, can affect or change your skin color throughout your life, but the inherent color of your skin is the result of those two pigments.

Eumelanin pigments are brown to black, so the higher their concentration, the deeper your skin tone. The less eumelanin you have, the more the white connective tissue underneath your dermis shines through and the lighter your complexion appears. Without eumelanin, skin is almost see-through, which is why veins and flushing are so much more visible in people with fair skin.

Eumelanin

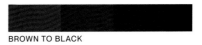

BROWN TO BLACK

Pheomelanin

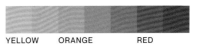

YELLOW   ORANGE   RED

While eumelanin determines the depth of your skin tone, its undertone depends on the amount and specific hue of its pheomelanin pigments, which can range from yellow to red. The more orange pheomelanin your skin contains, the warmer it will appear.

In the next few pages, we will look at some examples of cool to warm undertones across a spectrum of skin tones. Use the images to get a feel for how warmth (and a lack of it) shows up in the skin and see how your own complexion compares. Make sure to base your judgment solely on your facial skin. Disregard areas that are more pigmented due to dryness, such as around your mouth, and also ignore any redness that appears locally (such as on your cheeks).

This is how the amount of warmth you can detect in your skin translates to your skin's undertone:

- ☐ COOL UNDERTONE: (Almost) no warmth
- ☐ COOL-NEUTRAL: A little warmth
- ☐ WARM-NEUTRAL: Some warmth
- ☐ WARM: Obvious warmth

All skin tones contain a mix of every shade of pheomelanin, but the specific ratio will be unique to you and determine the hue of your skin. Of course, how that hue shows up also depends on your skin's eumelanin content. The chart opposite is an approximation of the hues you may be able to spot in different skin tones, depending on their dominant shade of pheomelanin. Note how your skin may also contain little of any kind of pheomelanin, in which case it will appear quite desaturated.

ADVANCED COLOR THEORY
Why your eye color does not reflect your undertone

Although your eye color is also determined by eumelanin, your eyes do not contain pheomelanin. In that sense, they cannot be "warm" or "cool," and their color is not correlated with the warmth of your skin and hair (as opposed to, for example, someone whose skin contains more pheomelanin also being likely to have hair that contains more pheomelanin). There are just as many warm-toned as cool-toned folks whose eyes are an icy blue, because the color of our eyes is a consequence of eumelanin—it has nothing to do with pheomelanin.

	Yellow	Orange	Red	Little of Any Kind
Dominant pheomelanin				
Hue of skin	OLIVE	RICH CHESTNUT TO PALE APRICOT	MAHOGANY TO SIENNA	DESATURATED
Undertone	COOL OR COOL-NEUTRAL	WARM OR WARM-NEUTRAL	COOL OR COOL-NEUTRAL	COOL OR COOL-NEUTRAL

YOUR UNDERTONE

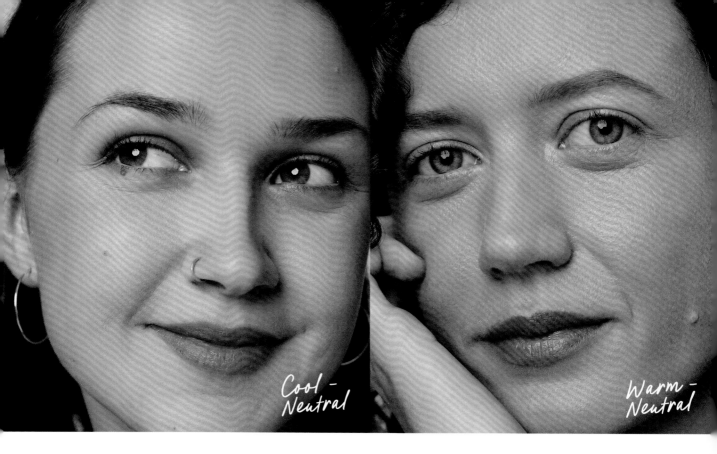

Cool-Neutral

Warm-Neutral

Compare Anastasia (left) and Theresa (right): Despite their fair skin tone, there is a clear difference in the amount of orange we can spot in their skin. Theresa's complexion is a pale gold with a warm-neutral undertone. Anastasia's skin also contains a little warmth: her undertone is cool-neutral.

Warmth in skin is orange

The more orange pheomelanin your skin contains, the warmer it will appear. Orange pheomelanin can range from a mango shade (a yellow-orange) to a papaya shade (a reddish orange). How that orange warmth shows up in the skin depends on its depth. Deeper warm skin tones may have a rich chestnut or tawny hue. In medium skin tones, warmth can appear as a golden ocher hue or an amber shade. Lighter warm skin tones have a paler golden tint or a more apricot hue. These hues are quite pronounced and easy to spot in skin with a warm undertone. In warm-neutral skin, they are more subtle but still clearly present once you know what to look for. Cool-neutral skin will also contain minor hints of warmth (see Anastasia, above left).

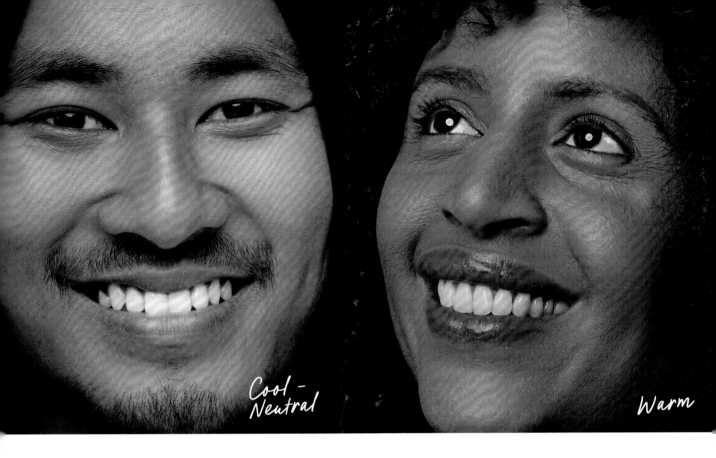

Cool – Neutral

Warm

Warmth in skin is orange, not yellow. Take a look at Okkar (left) and Yvonne (right): Both skin tones contain a high amount of yellow, but while Okkar's skin has an olive hue, Yvonne's skin has an orangey tinge. Okkar has a cool-neutral skin tone and Yvonne has a warm skin tone.

A yellow or olive tint is not a sign of warmth

If your skin has a yellow or olive tint to it, your skin cells may contain a higher concentration of yellow pheomelanin, which does not contribute to warmth. Remember: A color's undertone depends on how it compares to other shades of the same hue. Since human skin always contains some yellow, orange, and red pheomelanin, all skin tones are a part of the orange hue family. And the closer an orange shade gets to yellow, the cooler it gets.

Cool skin is defined by a lack of warmth

Your skin does not contain blue, purple, pink, or ashy pigments—it either contains a lot of orange pheomelanin, or it contains very little, in which case it will appear cool. There are two types of cool skin. The first type is cool because it contains very little pheomelanin of any kind and will, therefore, look quite desaturated and "ashy." This type of cool is more common in light and fair skin tones. The second type of cool skin does contain pheomelanin, but it is either the yellow or red kind, not the orange pheomelanin that adds warmth. Skin with a lot of yellow pheomelanin is commonly referred to as "olive" (more on page 112). Skin tones dominant in red pheomelanin are usually medium or deeper and may appear sienna or mahogany in color (like Zondy's skin on the right).

Pink skin is not necessarily cool

It's a misconception that redness or pink skin is an indicator of a cool undertone. If the pinkness of your skin appears only locally, it's not actually a result of the pigmentation in your dermis, but rather due to flushing, rosacea, or another skin sensitivity. If you have fair skin that has a subtle pink tinge all over and no visible amount of warmth, you may well have a cool undertone. But pink cheeks or local skin redness have nothing to do with your undertone.

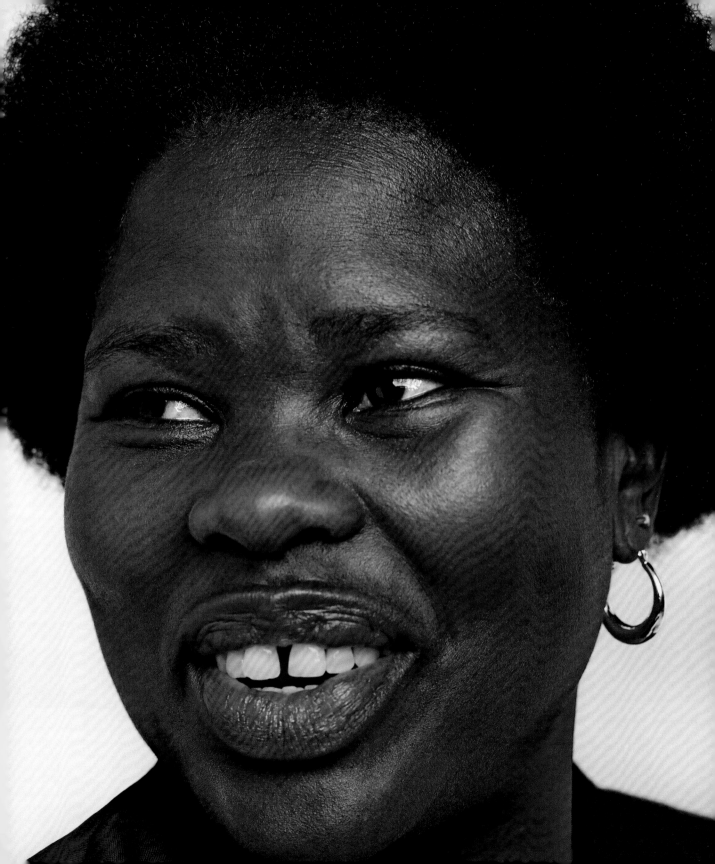

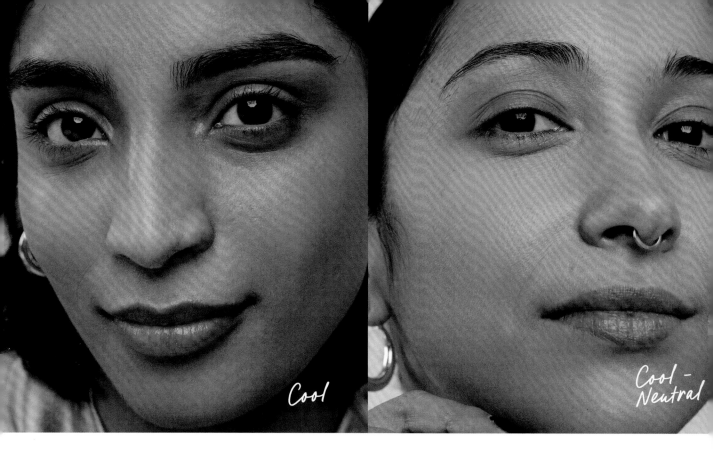

Cool

Cool – Neutral

Olive skin

If your skin appears olive, your skin cells contain a high concentration of yellow pheomelanin. When you mix that yellow with black eumelanin, you get a greenish hue that could also be called olive. Strictly speaking, olive skin is not actually olive (a green hue), since green hues are a mix of yellow and blue. It's a deep yellow.

It is a misconception that an olive hue indicates a warm undertone. Olive skin can appear richly yellow, golden, or bronzed—all terms that are commonly associated with warmth. But as mentioned on page 109, in skin, a yellow tint by itself is not a sign of warmth. Just like all skin tones, the more orange pheomelanin olive skin contains, the warmer its undertone.

Cool olive skin has a yellow hue that clearly leans green, as opposed to orange, and may appear somewhat desaturated. Cool-neutral

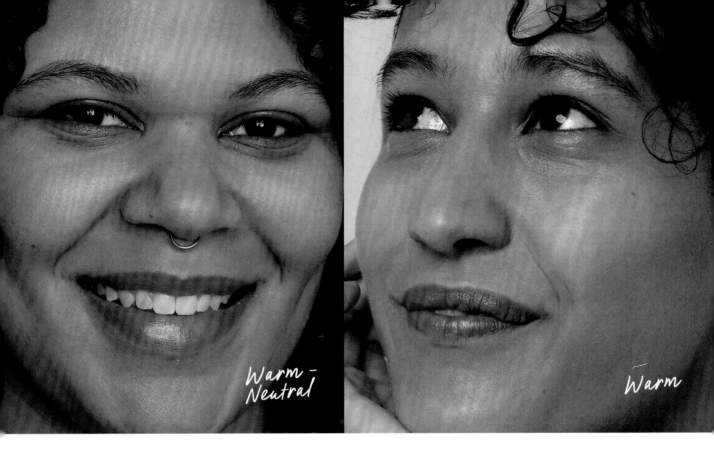

Warm - Neutral

Warm

olive skin will have a subtler green-ish tint. Cool-neutral is the most common undertone in olive skin tones. When in doubt, pick this category. For olive skin to have a warm undertone, your skin must contain high amounts of both yellow and orange pigments. All of that pheomelanin means your skin will be quite saturated (like the two photos above).

In this example, I've chosen models with similar (medium) skin tones to better illustrate how cool and warm olive complexions differ in tone. But any skin tone, from rich-deep to fair, can be olive.

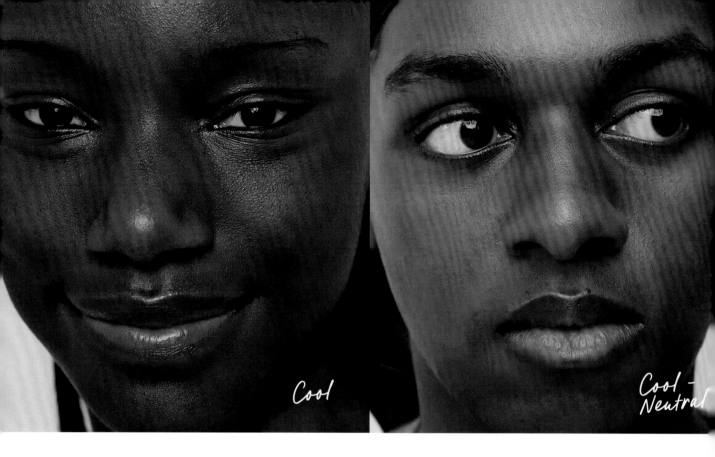

Cool

Cool - Neutral

Undertone in rich-deep, deep, and medium-deep skin tones

Deeper skin tones can have any undertone, with the exception that rich-deep skin is less likely to have a warm undertone (not warm-neutral). The deeper a color is, the smaller its chromatic component, and the closer it comes to a grayscale shade, which is cool. Black is 100 percent cool because it contains no warmth.

Deeper skin tones can be cool in three ways: they may have an olive hue that shows up as a deep bronze shade; they may appear a desaturated color like espresso or tobacco; or they may be dominant in red pheomelanin, giving the complexion a mahogany or russet shade.

Cool-neutral deeper skin will either be subtly olive or a balanced brown shade that appears to lean neither red nor orange.

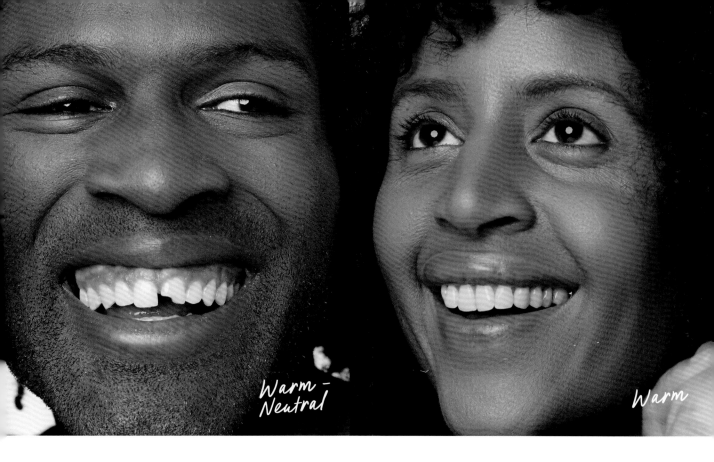

Warm - Neutral

Warm

Warm-neutral deeper skin will have subtle hints of a richer orange shade, such as copper or cinnamon. Warm skin tones contain more than just a subtle hint of these and tend to be quite saturated, leaning toward a deep orange hue, such as a rich chestnut or tawny.

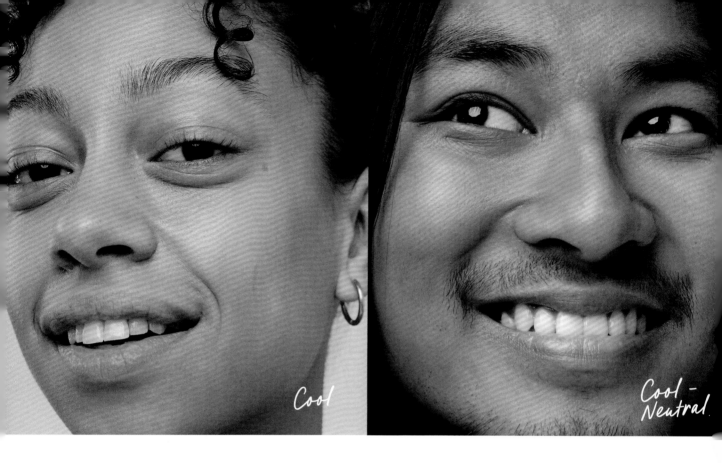

Cool

Cool – Neutral

Undertone in medium and light-medium skin tones

Medium and light-medium skin can have undertones ranging from cool to warm. Olive skin is common.

Cool medium or light-medium skin tones may have an obvious olive tint (without any warmth) or be relatively desaturated. Any yellow pigment in your skin will lean green, not orange. If your skin is obviously olive or desaturated but not totally devoid of orange warmth, your undertone may be cool-neutral—the most common undertone category across skin tones.

Medium skin tones (not light-medium) may also be dominant in red pheomelanin, resulting in sienna or clay hues. In this case,

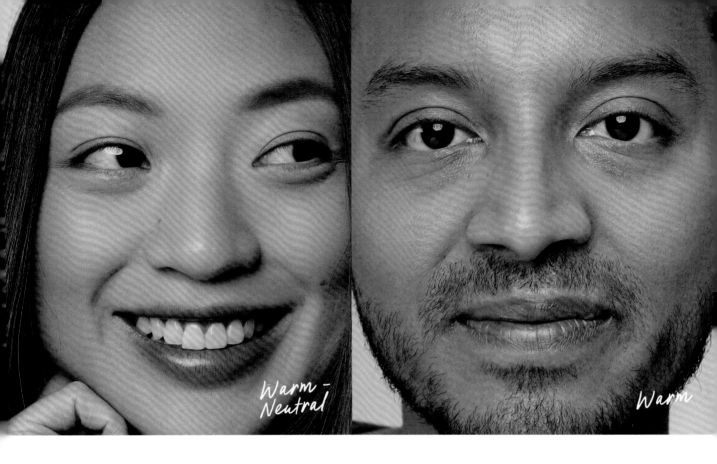

Warm – Neutral

Warm

their undertone will be cool or cool-neutral, depending on how pronounced the red tint is.

Medium or light-medium skin tones with a warm undertone radiate in shades of caramel, tawny, ocher, or ginger. Warm-neutral skin will contain hints of these.

Olive medium or light-medium skin tones that are warm-neutral or warm will contain high amounts of both yellow and orange pheomelanin, making their skin tone appear quite saturated. See page 113 for an example.

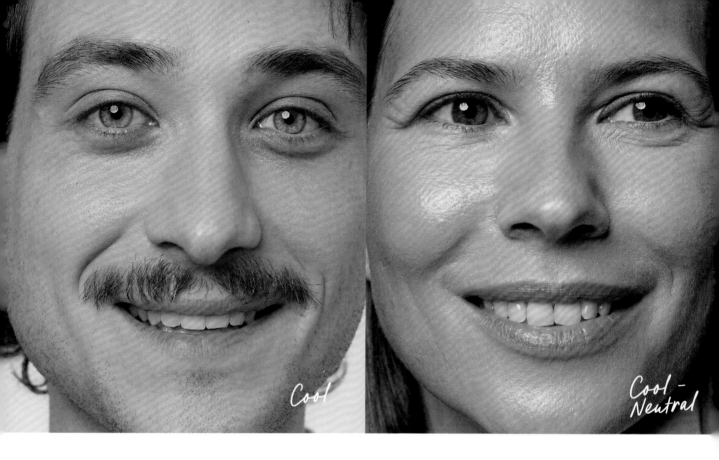

Cool

Cool – Neutral

Undertone in light and fair skin tones

Light and fair skin tones are often mistakenly considered to have a cool undertone, when in reality they are just as likely to be cool as they are to be warm-toned.

Olive skin is common in light skin, but rarer in fair skin. If your light or fair skin appears olive, its undertone is either cool or cool-neutral. Your skin is too light to contain both yellow and orange pheomelanin and still appear olive.

If your skin looks desaturated, ashy, or has a pink tinge, it may have very little pheomelanin, indicating a cool undertone. Cool-neutral skin contains a small amount of warmth and comes closest to what many people think of as a "neutral" undertone. If you believe your skin has

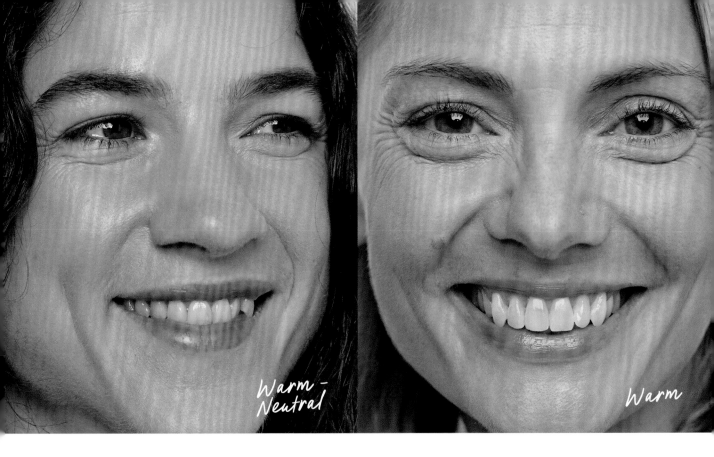

Warm - Neutral

Warm

a truly neutral undertone, it is likely cool-neutral. Warm lighter skin tones can range from a golden apricot shade to a peachy hue. For a warm undertone, your skin needs to visibly contain orange warmth. Otherwise, it is likely warm-neutral.

If you have freckles, you're in luck, because they can tell you a lot about your undertone! People with a warm or warm-neutral undertone will have almost orange freckles, while freckles on cool complexions will be a grayish brown shade.

Undertone in hair

Just like your skin tone, the color and undertone of your hair is determined by its unique ratio of eumelanin and pheomelanin pigments. Brown-black eumelanin pigments determine the depth of your hair, and orange pheomelanin pigments determine its warmth. Brown and black hair contain a lot of both types of melanin. Red hair contains more pheomelanin. Light blond hair contains small amounts of both types, but a large part of the off-white color of the hair's keratin shows through. Gray hair is also the result of that keratin color with some leftover eumelanin.

Compared to your skin tone, your natural hair color is a far less reliable marker of your overall undertone. That is because most natural hair colors are quite desaturated, which means their chromatic component is small, making any warmth hard to spot. Many people with a warm skin tone have hair that doesn't seem to contain a lot of warmth, but their hair may simply be too desaturated, light, or deep for warmth to show up. Because of that, we will not count the absence of warmth in your hair as an indicator that your overall coloring is cool. On the other hand, if there is warmth in your hair, we will remember that, and at the end of the chapter we will combine it with the evidence we have collected on your skin tone.

Ignore facial hair when determining your undertone

For many people, facial hair, specifically beards, can have a considerably warmer undertone than the hair on their head. This mismatch is a rare exception to one of the key principles of color harmony and color analysis: that our natural coloring is innately congruent. Usually, someone whose skin contains more pheomelanin is also more likely to have hair that contains more pheomelanin (on both their face and head). That is why we can draw conclusions about your overall undertone by assessing your hair and skin tone separately. But if the hair in your beard region is considerably more red-toned than the hair on your head, we cannot use it as an indicator for your undertone, because its hue is entirely unrelated to the rest of your melanin formula.

The amount of pheomelanin in our skin and hair is regulated by one specific gene, *MC1R*. Among many other things, *MC1R* causes pheomelanin to be converted to eumelanin. People with red hair of any kind have a mutation in both copies of that gene, causing less pheomelanin to get converted. It is believed that in people whose facial hair has a warmer undertone than the hair on their head, only one copy of the *MC1R* gene is mutated, which, curiously, seems to be reflected mainly in a person's facial hair.

How much warmth does your natural hair color contain?

Use the examples on the next few pages to determine whether your natural hair color contains no warmth (or almost none), some warmth, or obvious warmth. Ignore any bits of your hair that seem warmer and lighter than the rest, such as the ends, finer hairs around your hairline, and any "natural highlights." Even if you have not colored your hair, certain bits may have gotten bleached by the sun. Hair inevitably warms up whenever it gets bleached, whether chemically or through sun exposure. That is because the orange pheomelanin pigments are more resistant to bleach and UV exposure than the brown-black eumelanin pigments.

(Almost) no warmth

If your natural hair color comes close to the following, you likely won't be able to spot any warmth in your hair.

Black or black-brown (Hair levels 1–2)

Hair that is very deep toned is too densely packed with eumelanin for any pheomelanin to be visible. That does not mean your strands don't contain any pheomelanin; they do, otherwise they'd look charcoal, rather than black or black-brown.

Espresso or chocolate brown (Hair levels 3–5)

Brown hair does not need to look "ashy" to qualify as cool. If your hair is a medium to deep brown and you cannot spot any hints of gold, amber, or bronze near the crown (not the ends), this is your level. Important: Subtle reddish highlights that show up under certain lighting are not a sign of warmth! The warmth we are looking for has an orange hue.

Cool brown to ash blond (Hair levels 6+)

Lighter hair that contains (almost) no warmth looks ashy and desaturated. If you are a level 8 blond or above, your hair likely contains at least some warmth.

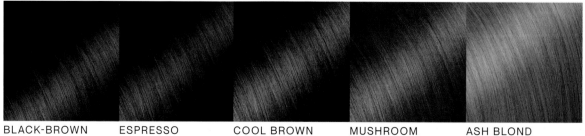

BLACK-BROWN   ESPRESSO   COOL BROWN   MUSHROOM BROWN   ASH BLOND

Some warmth

There are three groups of natural hair colors that contain some but not obvious warmth.

Warm brown (Hair levels 4–7)

Is your hair level 4 to 7 brown with an obvious bronzy, amber, or golden hue? If your shade of brown can be described as cinnamon or golden, pick this category.

Auburn (Hair level 4)

Auburn hair is a level 4 with an obvious red tint. Auburn hair contains "some warmth" rather than "obvious warmth," because the red in auburn hair is quite a bit cooler than the orange hue that characterizes warmth.

Medium to light blond (Hair levels 8+)

Many blonds mislabel their hair as "ashy" when it is simply very light. If your hair is a level 8 or above and has even the faintest yellowish hue, it contains at least some pheomelanin. Otherwise, it would just look gray.

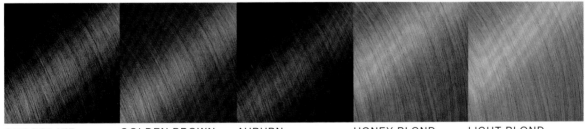

CHOCOLATE BROWN GOLDEN BROWN AUBURN HONEY BLOND LIGHT BLOND

Obvious warmth

Hair with obvious warmth has a strong orange or golden (that is, yellow) tinge. These types of colors are relatively rare and more common at medium to lighter hair levels, because a high concentration of eumelanin would cover up all that warmth. If your hair color comes close to the following, it contains obvious warmth.

Titian or deep red (Hair levels 5–6)

If your level 5 or 6 hair has a strong red-orange hue, it has obvious warmth.

Red, copper, or strawberry blond (Hair levels 6–10)

If your natural hair color is red at a hair level 6 to 10, it contains obvious warmth. Case closed. This includes all types of strawberry blond.

Golden light brown or honey blond (Hair levels 7–9)

For non-red hair to fall into the "obvious warmth" category, it needs to be relatively light (hair level 7 and above) and have an obvious yellow hue, like a golden light brown or honey blond. Very light blond hair (level 10) is usually not warm enough.

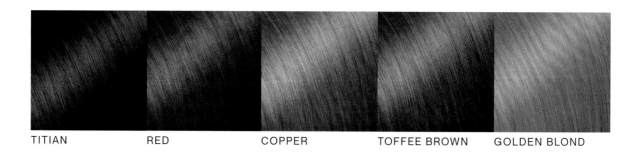

TITIAN   RED   COPPER   TOFFEE BROWN   GOLDEN BLOND

What is your undertone?

Now it's time to put together all the information you have collected and determine your overall undertone. Use this table to see where your evidence puts you. Which two categories best fit your coloring's overall undertone: cool, cool-neutral, warm-neutral or warm?

		Hair		
		NO WARMTH	A LITTLE WARMTH	OBVIOUS WARMTH
Skin	COOL	cool	cool-neutral	*check again*
	COOL-NEUTRAL	cool-neutral	warm-neutral	warm-neutral
	WARM-NEUTRAL	warm-neutral	warm-neutral	warm
	WARM	warm	warm	warm

Your turn

- ☐ Determine your skin's undertone by assessing its level of orange warmth. If you have olive skin, make sure you are not mistaking a yellow hue for warmth.

- ☐ Gather bonus evidence by checking if your hair color contains warmth.

- ☐ Combine your evidence to choose two out of the four undertone categories.

YOUR CHROMA

Soft, Medium, or Clear?

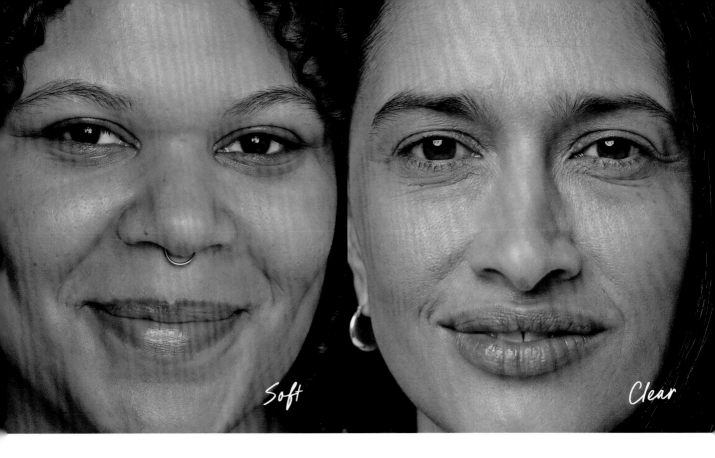

Soft

Clear

Dugga (left) and Diana (right) both have a medium skin tone with a warm-neutral undertone and dark brown hair, but their coloring is quite different, isn't it? Dugga's complexion has a muted, blended appearance, while Diana's skin is more saturated. Dugga's eyes are a deep black-brown, while Diana's eyes are a vivid red-brown.

CATEGORIES: soft, medium, or clear

RELEVANT FEATURES: Skin tone and eye color

Your chroma depends on the inherent vibrancy and saturation of your skin tone and eye color. People with high chroma naturally have a lot of brightness in their coloring and are able to pull off bolder, more saturated shades. Those same shades would overwhelm someone with low chroma, who has a gentler, softer coloring that is complemented by a more muted, desaturated color palette. Your chroma may also be medium: in that case, you can handle some color intensity, but very vivid shades will likely overwhelm you. All skin tones can be soft, medium, or clear. Keep in mind, your chroma is also independent of your contrast level.

Chroma is the most elusive aspect of our color trio—hard to figure out and easy to misinterpret. Compared to your contrast level and undertone, determining your chroma requires a much more holistic assessment of your coloring. How bright and saturated does your face appear as a whole (without makeup or any sort of tan)? How vivid is your eye color? Do you have natural blushing? Are your lips on the paler end or more rosy? Do you have freckles? In this chapter, we will determine your chroma based on two factors: your skin tone and eye color. Since human hair is generally desaturated, the color of your strands is not a good indicator of your chroma, so your hair can sit this one out.

Remember that you do not need to figure out your exact chroma at this stage. Aim to determine which two of the three chroma categories best fit your coloring: soft, medium, or clear.

Chroma in skin

As we know, chroma tells us how "full of color" a shade is, how much of its hue it has, and how much of it is a grayscale shade. Compare this magenta shade at different levels of chroma. The higher the chroma, the more vivid and clear it looks. The lower the chroma, the more gray is mixed in, and the more muted and soft the shade looks. Important: Only gray is an indicator of low chroma; black and white are not! If we mix a pure magenta hue with a lot of white, we will get a bright, high-chroma pastel pink. If we mix a pure magenta hue with

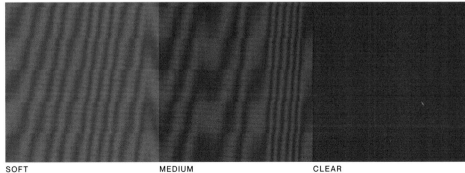

SOFT   MEDIUM   CLEAR

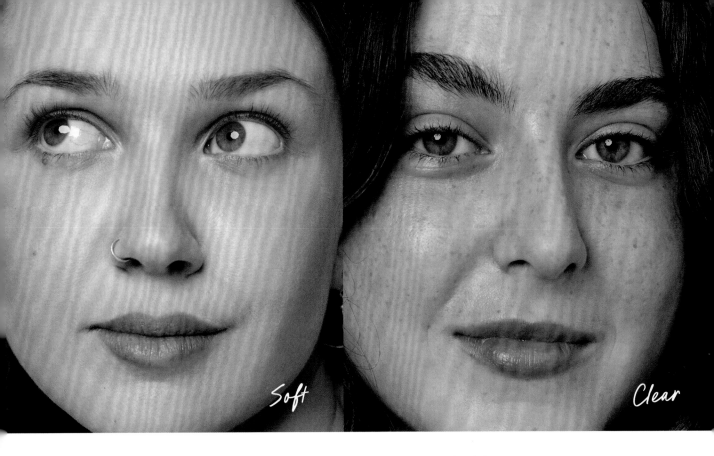

Soft

Clear

Compare Anastasia (left) and Elisa (right) above: Both have a fair skin tone, but Anastasia's coloring seems a lot softer and more delicate than Elisa's, who has a ton of built-in color intensity with her freckles, bright eyes, and saturated lips.

black, we will get an intense shade of blackberry. The chroma of a shade is all about how much gray it contains.

But what does skin with a high chroma look like? Can skin also look vivid or more muted? Yes! Just like any other shade, the color of your skin can be saturated or more desaturated, and we can determine its chroma by assessing how much gray it contains.

Soft chroma skin contains quite a lot of gray and will appear visibly muted. You will have very little natural blushing, if any, and your lips will be a similar color to your skin. Regardless of your skin tone, you may sometimes feel like your skin looks pale or "tired." Clear chroma skin contains almost no gray and appears luminous and bright. Regardless of your skin tone, your complexion does not look pale, sallow, or "dull." If you are somewhere in the middle, your skin likely has a medium chroma.

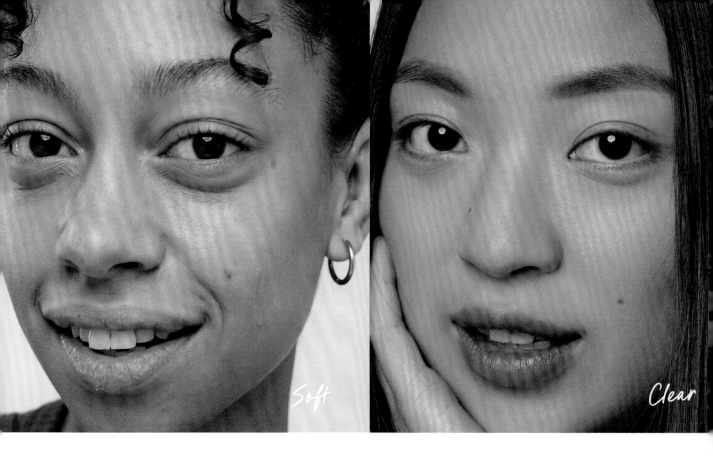

Soft

Clear

In my experience, deep skin tones are more likely to have clear or medium chroma. In lighter and medium skin tones, all chroma categories are equally common. Compare Camille (left) and Jülly (right): Can you see how Jülly's complexion has more color intensity overall, while Camille's complexion appears more blended and muted?

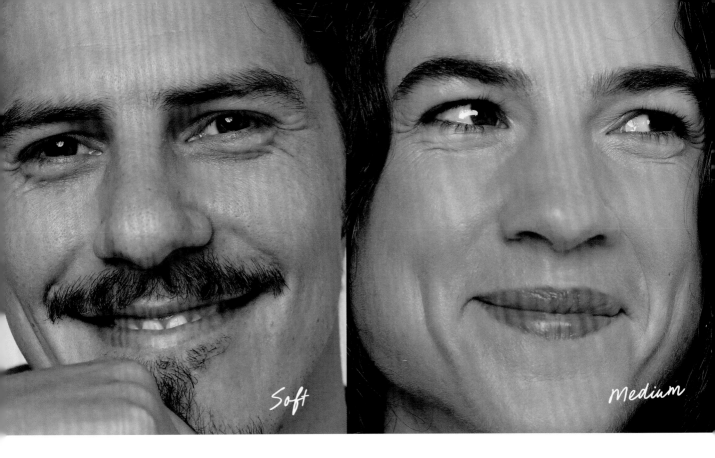

Soft

Medium

Next, compare Iason (left) and Sarah (right): Both have light skin, but Sarah's higher chroma skin has a brighter golden hue, while Iason's lower chroma skin is more subdued. Remember that, as far as colors go, human skin is generally low chroma, so the difference between high-chroma and low-chroma skin will always be comparatively small.

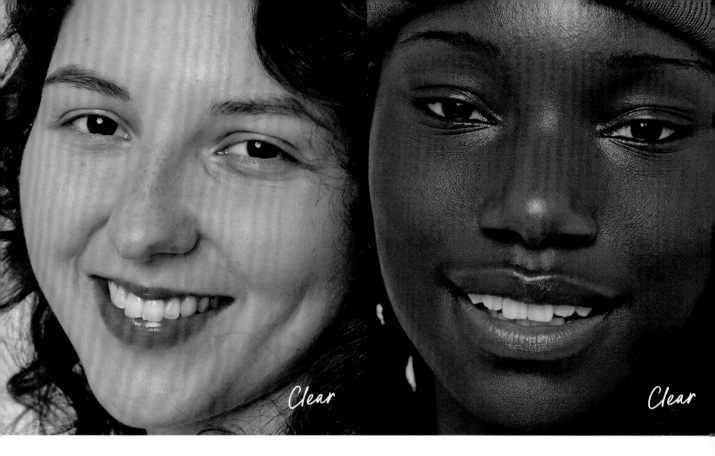

Clear

Clear

High chroma is characterized by a lack of gray

I recommend you determine your skin's chroma by assessing how much gray you can spot, rather than how "colorful" it appears. That is because if you look for saturation directly, you'll likely underestimate the chroma of both deep and fair skin tones. Rich-deep, deep, and fair skin will never contain a lot of color, but it's just as likely to have a high chroma as medium skin tones. Do you see how Tori's skin (on the left) is very fair and not "saturated," but it contains absolutely no hints of gray or ashiness? It is very clear. The same goes for Selena's rich-deep skin tone (on the right): there is not a lot of color per se, but it's undoubtedly very clear, because there is no gray. Remember: As colors, both black and white have a high chroma, because they contain no gray.

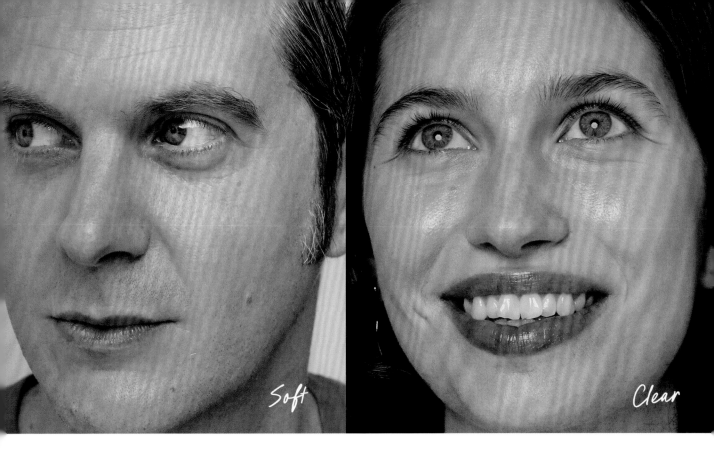

Soft

Clear

Do not mistake coolness for softness

Cool skin tones (especially light and fair ones) often contain very little pheomelanin, which can make your skin appear desaturated, much like a low chroma would. But cool skin is just as likely to be clear as soft. Compare Aristos (left) and Tordis (right), who both have almost no warmth in their skin and a cool undertone. Aristos's skin has a pale rose shade and appears subdued and gentle. Tordis's complexion has an alabaster tone; it's luminous and bright. The difference may seem subtle, but the impact on their best colors is considerable. Aristos's soft chroma means that cool, vivid shades like lapis blue, hot pink, and also black and white will overwhelm his delicate complexion. On Tordis those same shades will look effortless and natural.

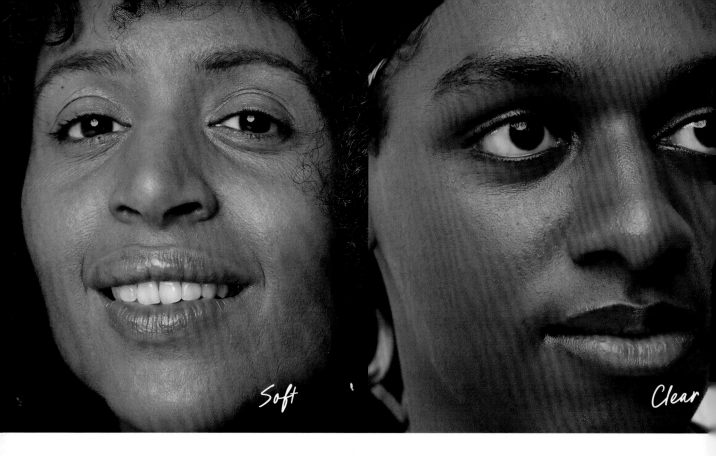

Soft

Clear

Chroma in rich-deep, deep, and medium-deep skin tones

Deeper skin tones tend to have clearer chromas than medium or lighter skin tones, because the deeper your skin tone, the smaller the chromatic component that could be gray. If your skin tone is rich-deep, your chroma is likely clear, possibly medium, but not soft. If your skin tone is deep or medium-deep, ask yourself whether your skin comes closer to a muted gray-brown shade or a richer brown hue like mahogany or chestnut. If you cannot spot any gray, and your skin appears obviously saturated, luminous, and bright, your chroma is clear. If your skin tone is neither very saturated nor gray-based, your chroma is likely medium. For deeper skin to be considered soft, it needs to appear clearly desaturated and muted, like Yvonne's (left). You will not have any natural blushing, and your lips will be comparatively pale.

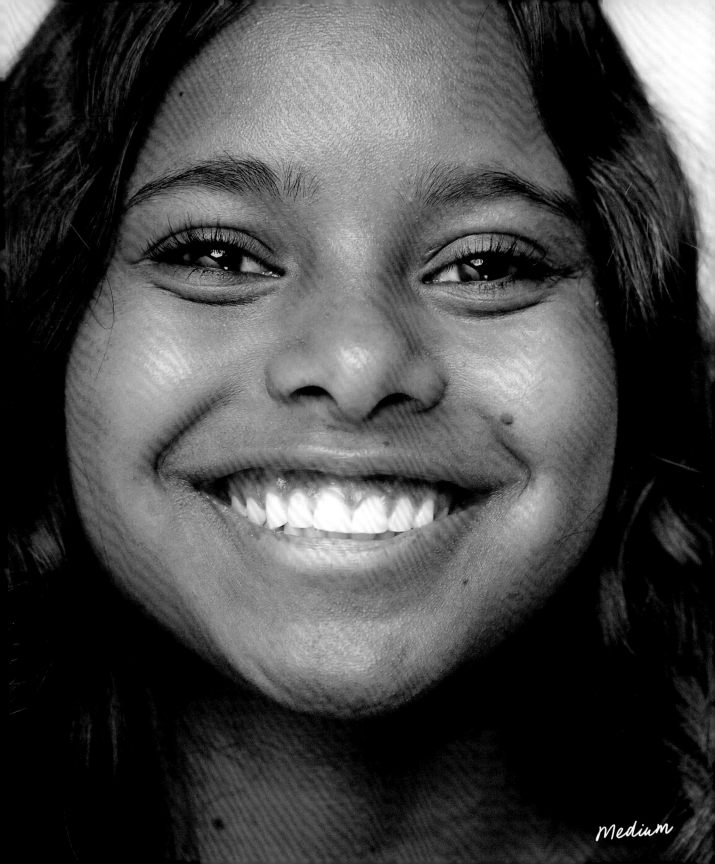

Medium

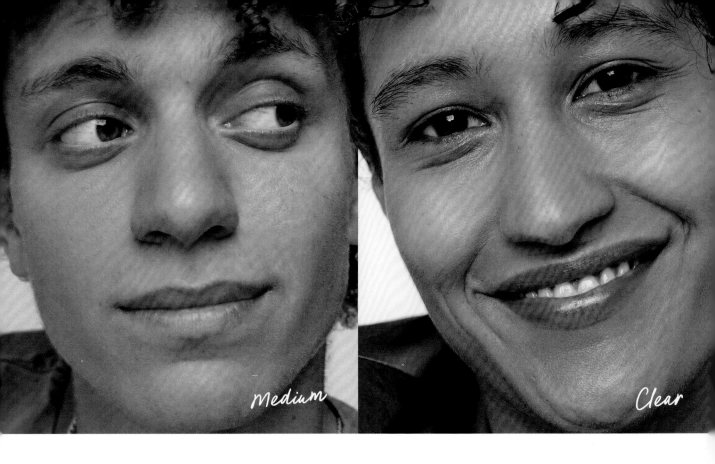

Medium

Clear

Chroma in medium and light-medium skin tones

Your skin tone is just as likely to be soft as it is clear. Compare the saturation of your skin to the models above: Is your skin tone radiant and saturated like Rachel's (above right)? Or more gray-based and subdued like Graciela's (opposite)? Or perhaps somewhere in the middle like Amin's (above left)? Can you spot any high-chroma markers such as natural blushing, rosy lips, or freckles?

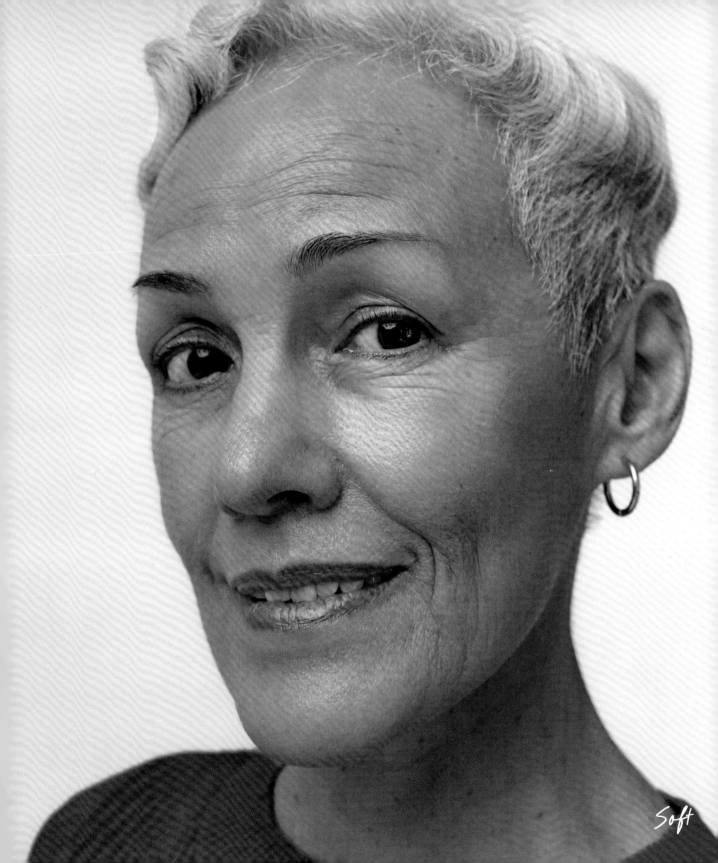

Soft

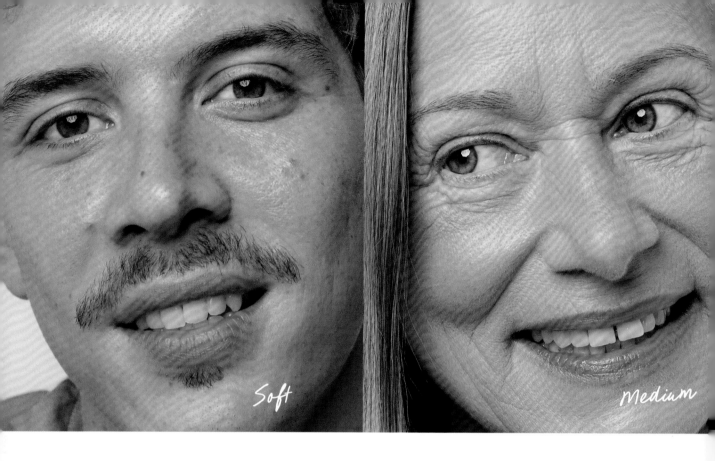

Soft

Medium

Chroma in lighter skin tones

Light and fair skin tones are equally likely to have a soft, medium, and clear chroma, but the lighter your skin the trickier it can be to detect the saturation of your skin tone. While you can and should assess the chroma of your skin the same way you would evaluate the chroma of any color (by looking for saturation versus gray), there are additional markers that often go hand in hand with a high chroma in light and fair skin tones: natural flushing, rosy lips, and freckles. All of these add extra color intensity and luminosity to your face as a whole.

None of these are needed to qualify as clear. If your skin tone appears saturated, that is all the information you need.

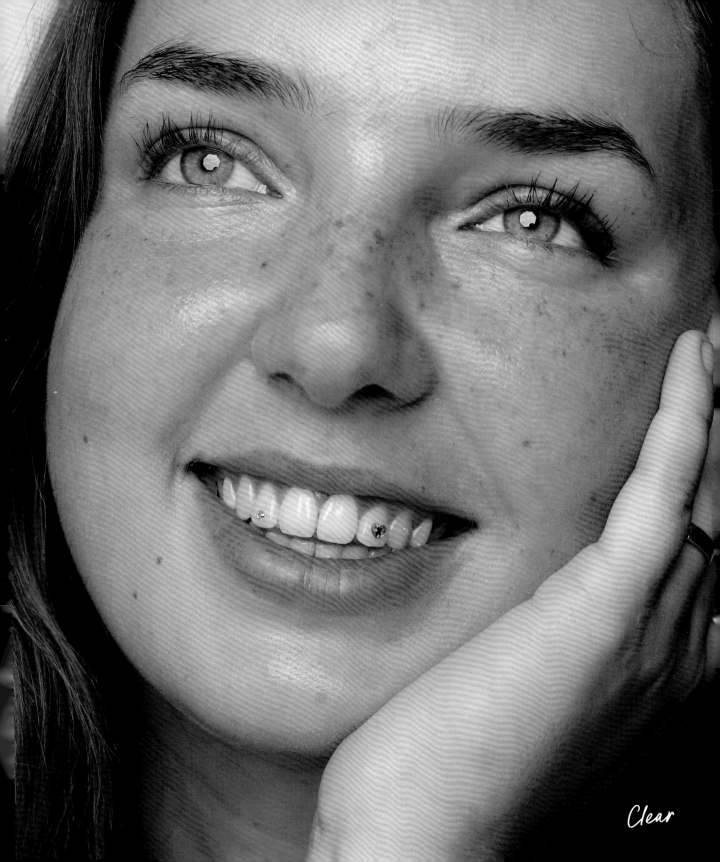

Clear

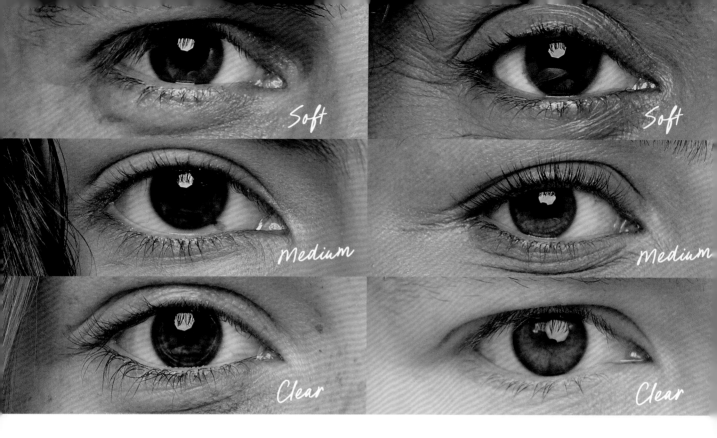

Soft

Soft

Medium

Medium

Clear

Clear

Chroma in eyes

Unlike hair colors, the chroma spectrum of human eye colors is vast, and someone's eye color can often provide additional evidence for their overall chroma. The best way to gauge the chroma of your eyes depends on their hue. Refer back to page 90 if you are not sure how to classify your exact eye color.

Black-brown eyes

If your eyes are a deep brown or black, you likely won't be able to spot any red or yellow in them. Although this is not an indication that the chroma of your overall coloring is low, you unfortunately can't use your eye color to determine your overall chroma.

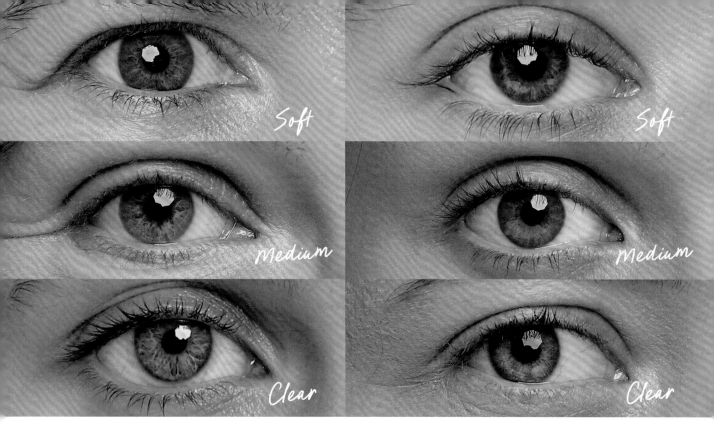

Soft

Soft

Medium

Medium

Clear

Clear

Brown and hazel eyes

If you have brown eyes, the more red or yellow you can find, the clearer your eyes are. Softer brown eyes have more of a gray-brown hue. Clear brown eyes are a saturated amber or rust shade, medium-chroma brown eyes are brown with a more subtle golden or red tint. Since hazel eyes are essentially lighter, higher-chroma browns, they are never soft. Clear hazel eyes are vivid golden brown; medium-chroma hazel eyes are light brown with a green tint.

Green, blue, and gray eyes

If you have green, blue, or gray eyes, determine how far your eyes are from a medium gray. Blue or green eyes with a clear chroma will be either vivid or quite light and icy. Soft eyes of this type are more desaturated and deeper: If your eyes are a grayish or blue-green shade that you never quite know what to call, chances are your eyes are soft.

What is your overall chroma?

Use the table below to select up to two chroma categories that best fit your overall chroma. If your eyes are black-brown, you will need to choose your two most likely chroma categories based on your complexion alone.

Remember that chroma is the most elusive color dimension! Unless your chroma is very pronounced, you may not feel too confident about your result. That is okay, because we are going to treat your chroma as only an estimate at this stage. We are not using it to exclude any seasons, just to select a short list of potential seasons that you'll test out during the draping stage.

	Eyes	SOFT	MEDIUM	CLEAR
Complexion	SOFT	soft	soft	medium
	MEDIUM	medium	medium	clear
	CLEAR	check again	clear	clear

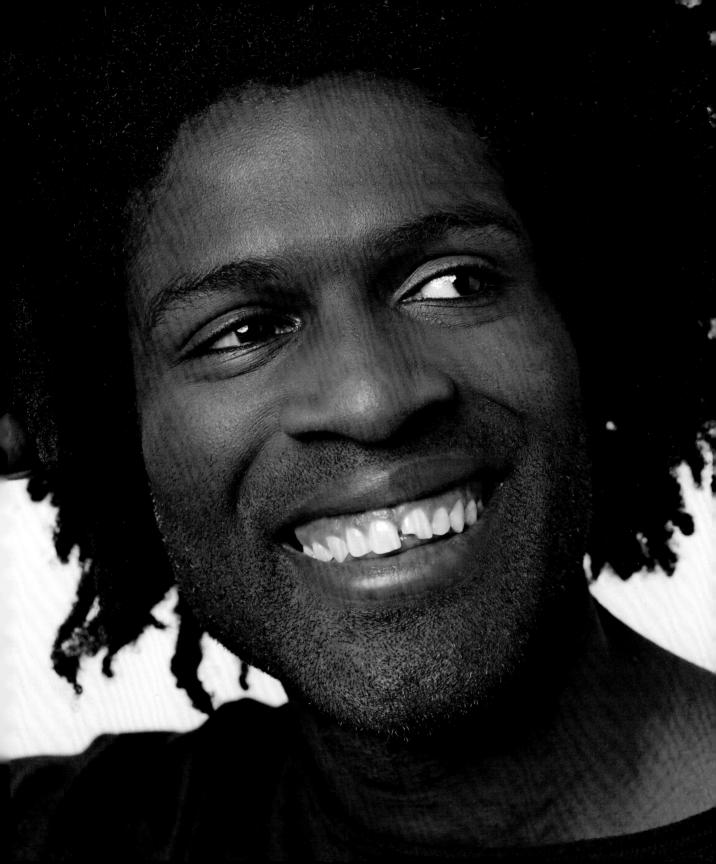

DRAPING

How to Confirm Your Season by Testing Out Colors

Now that you have analyzed your coloring from all angles and estimated your contrast level, undertone, and chroma, you are one step closer to finding your season. But you are not ready to commit to one type yet. Your most likely matches need to pass one last round: the draping. In color analysis, a drape is any fabric that you can hold up to your face to see how well a specific color harmonizes with your coloring. Only once you have tried out a season's colors in real life and compared it to related seasons can you claim a season as "the one." This chapter will walk you through exactly how to do that.

What are your most likely seasons?

If you go to a professional color analyst, they will likely sit you down in front of a mirror and drape you in a whole range of colors. They will cast a wide net, covering all undertones, values, and chromas, so that they can slowly work their way toward your most harmonious colors. But *you* won't need to test nearly as many colors during your at-home draping session, because you have already done a lot of work to home in on your season. Using the information you have gathered about your contrast level, undertone, and chroma, you can now select three to six seasons as your most likely matches and focus on them during the draping stage.

A quick recap: Each of the twelve color seasons corresponds to a specific combination of contrast, undertone, and chroma. For example, if your contrast level is medium, your undertone warm, and your chroma clear, your coloring matches the True Spring season.

Of course, at this stage, you likely do not feel 100 percent confident about your color dimensions. Perhaps you can say for certain that your contrast level is high or very high, and that your chroma is clear or medium. As for your undertone, maybe you think it's likely cool-neutral but can't exclude that it may be warm-neutral. You won't know your final color dimensions until *after* your draping session—after you've identified the one season with colors that harmonize the best with your coloring. Therefore, your next step is to identify all seasons that match any combination of the color dimensions you have estimated using the table on the following page.

Your closest match

Undertone	Chroma	Contrast			
		VERY HIGH	**HIGH**	**MEDIUM**	**LOW**
COOL	CLEAR	True Winter	True Winter	Could your undertone be cool-neutral? If yes, try Clear Winter.	Could your undertone be cool-neutral and your chroma medium? If yes, try Light Summer.
	MEDIUM	Could your chroma be clear? If yes, try True Winter.	Could your chroma be clear? If yes, try True Winter.	Could your chroma be soft? If yes, try True Summer.	Could your chroma be soft? If yes, try True Summer.
	SOFT	Could your undertone be cool-neutral and your contrast high? If yes, try Soft Summer.	Could your undertone be cool-neutral? If yes, try Soft Summer.	True Summer	True Summer
COOL-NEUTRAL	CLEAR	Could your undertone be cool? If yes, try True Winter.	Clear Winter	Clear Winter	Light Summer
	MEDIUM	Deep Winter	Deep Winter	Light Summer	Light Summer
	SOFT	Could your contrast be high? If yes, try Soft Summer.	Soft Summer	Soft Summer	Could your undertone be cool? If yes, try True Summer.
WARM-NEUTRAL	CLEAR	Could your contrast be high? If yes, try Clear Spring.	Clear Spring	Clear Spring	Could your undertone be warm? If yes, try Light Spring.
	MEDIUM	Deep Autumn	Deep Autumn	Light Spring	Light Spring
	SOFT	Could your undertone be warm? If yes, try True Autumn.	Soft Autumn	Soft Autumn	Could your undertone be warm? If yes, try Light Spring.
WARM	CLEAR	Could your undertone be warm-neutral and your contrast high? If yes, try Clear Spring.	Could your undertone be warm-neutral? If yes, try Clear Spring.	True Spring	True Spring
	MEDIUM	Could your undertone be warm-neutral? If yes, try Deep Autumn.	Could your undertone be warm-neutral? If yes, try Deep Autumn.	Could your chroma be clear? If yes, try True Spring.	Could your chroma be clear? If yes, try True Spring.
	SOFT	True Autumn	True Autumn	Could your undertone be warm-neutral? If yes, try Soft Autumn.	Could your undertone be warm-neutral and your chroma medium? If yes, try Light Spring.

In our example, if your undertone is indeed cool-neutral, there are two seasons that fit your likely chroma and contrast: Clear Winter (clear chroma, high contrast) and Deep Winter (medium chroma, high and very high contrast).

While no season matches the combination of a clear chroma and very high contrast, the table suggests trying True Winter if your undertone could be cool (instead of cool-neutral). But you can reject that suggestion since you are sure your undertone is either cool-neutral or warm-neutral. Otherwise, you would add True Winter to your shortlist as well.

Now let's check which seasons correspond to your criteria if your undertone is warm-neutral. According to the table, there are two: Clear Spring and Deep Autumn.

So, in total, you have four most likely seasons that you can focus on during the draping stage: Clear Winter, Deep Winter, Clear Spring, and Deep Autumn.

Depending on your dimensions, your short list will include anywhere from three to six seasons.

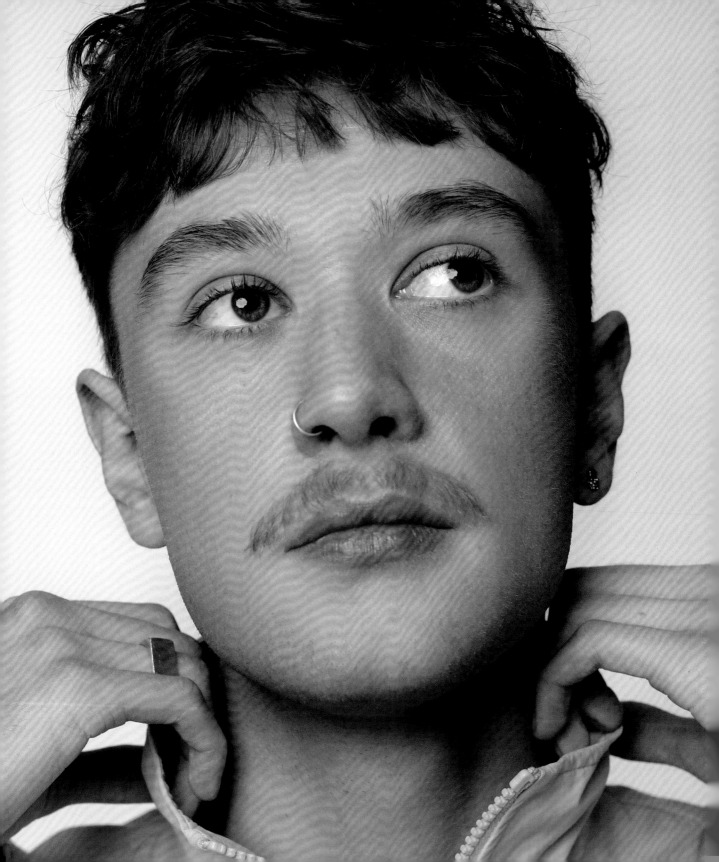

Which colors should you test out?

Depending on the number of seasons on your short list, you will need to drape fifteen to thirty colors. If that sounds like a lot, don't worry. We will discuss how to find all those drapes later on, but it's not as hard as you may think. For each season on your short list, I recommend you try on five colors:

☐ Two "classic" shades that represent that season's color palette and will obviously look good on anyone belonging to that season.

☐ Two uniquely harmonious shades that are hard to pull off for the majority of people, except for the people in that one season.

☐ One uniquely dissonant shade that tends to be generally flattering to most people, except for people belonging to that season.

You'll find an overview of the shades in the type profiles on the next page.

Are you a Clear Spring?

Test out these colors

1 Do these two shades
   work well on you?

TRUE RED   APPLE GREEN

2 Can you pull off these two
   hard-to-wear colors?

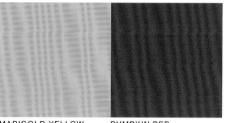

MARIGOLD YELLOW   PUMPKIN RED

3 Is this shade not
   your best?

TAUPE

Interpret your results

If you answered yes to all three questions
you are a Clear Spring!

If the first four shades look . . .

too cool and deep	→	try True Spring.
too warm	→	try Clear Winter.
too clear and light	→	try Deep Autumn.
too clear and deep	→	try Light Spring.

Are you a True Spring?

Test out these colors

1 Do these two shades
   work well on you?

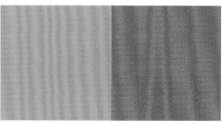

LIGHT OLIVE   PAPAYA

2 Can you pull off these two
   hard-to-wear colors?

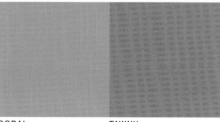

CORAL   TAWNY

3 Is this shade not
   your best?

DEEP STEEL BLUE

Interpret your results

If you answered yes to all three questions
you are a True Spring!

If the first four shades look . . .

too deep and clear	→	try Light Spring.
too light and warm	→	try Clear Spring.
too clear and light	→	try True Autumn.
too clear and soft	→	try Soft Autumn.

PERSONAL COLOR

Are you a Light Spring?

Test out these colors

1 Do these two shades work well on you?

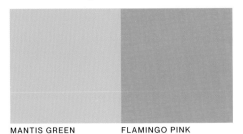

MANTIS GREEN   FLAMINGO PINK

2 Can you pull off these two hard-to-wear colors?

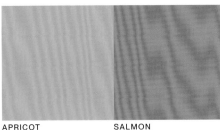

APRICOT   SALMON

3 Is this shade not your best?

CHARCOAL

Interpret your results

If you answered yes to all three questions you are a Light Spring!

If the first four shades look . . .

too light and cool	→	try True Spring.
too warm	→	try Light Summer.
too light and soft	→	try Clear Spring.
too clear and light	→	try Soft Autumn.

Are you a Light Summer?

Test out these colors

1 Do these two shades work well on you?

LIGHT BLUE   PARIS GREEN

2 Can you pull off these two hard-to-wear colors?

PALE ROSE   PALE AQUA

3 Is this shade not your best?

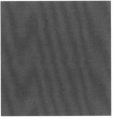

GOLDEN BROWN

Interpret your results

If you answered yes to all three questions you are a Light Summer!

If the first four shades look . . .

too cool	→	try Light Spring.
too light and warm	→	try True Summer.
too clear and light	→	try Soft Summer.

Are you a True Summer?

Test out these colors

1 Do these two shades work well on you?

CORN FLOWER   SKY MAGENTA

2 Can you pull off these two hard-to-wear colors?

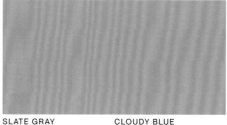

SLATE GRAY   CLOUDY BLUE

3 Is this shade not your best?

MARIGOLD YELLOW

Interpret your results

If you answered yes to all three questions you are a True Summer!

If the first four shades look . . .

too soft and deep	→	try Light Summer.
too clear and cool	→	try Soft Summer.
too soft	→	try True Winter.
too soft and cool	→	try Clear Winter.

Are you a Soft Summer?

Test out these colors

1 Do these two shades work well on you?

BOYSENBERRY   DUSKY TEAL

2 Can you pull off these two hard-to-wear colors?

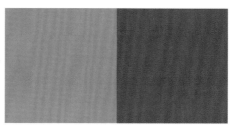

LAVENDER   ASH GRAY

3 Is this shade not your best?

NAPLES YELLOW

Interpret your results

If you answered yes to all three questions you are a Soft Summer!

If the first four shades look . . .

too warm	→	try True Summer.
too cool	→	try Soft Autumn.
too soft and deep	→	try Light Summer.
too soft and light	→	try Deep Winter.

Are you a Soft Autumn?

Test out these colors

1 Do these two shades work well on you?

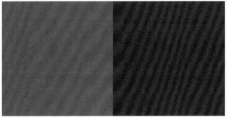

GREEN OLIVE   ROSEWOOD

2 Can you pull off these two hard-to-wear colors?

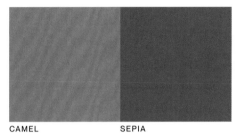

CAMEL   SEPIA

3 Is this shade not your best?

SHOCKING PINK

Interpret your results

If you answered yes to all three questions you are a Soft Autumn!

If the first four shades look . . .

too warm	→	try Soft Summer.
too cool	→	try True Autumn.
too deep and soft	→	try True Spring.
too light	→	try Deep Autumn.

Are you a True Autumn?

Test out these colors

1 Do these two shades work well on you?

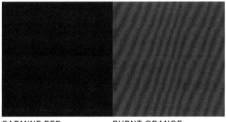

CARMINE RED   BURNT ORANGE

2 Can you pull off these two hard-to-wear colors?

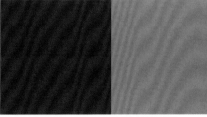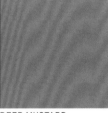

WARM BROWN   DEEP MUSTARD

3 Is this shade not your best?

PALE LILAC

Interpret your results

If you answered yes to all three questions you are a True Autumn!

If the first four shades look . . .

too warm and deep	→	try Soft Autumn.
too soft and light	→	try Deep Autumn.
too deep and soft	→	try True Spring.

Are you a Deep Autumn?

Test out these colors

1 Do these two shades work well on you?

BORDEAUX   PINE GREEN

2 Can you pull off these two hard-to-wear colors?

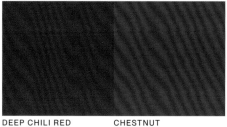

DEEP CHILI RED   CHESTNUT

3 Is this shade not your best?

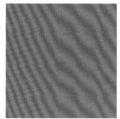

COOL PINK

Interpret your results

If you answered yes to all three questions you are a Deep Autumn!

If the first four shades look . . .

too clear and cool	→	try True Autumn.
too warm and soft	→	try Deep Winter.
too clear and deep	→	try Soft Autumn.
too soft and deep	→	try Clear Spring.

Are you a Deep Winter?

Test out these colors

1 Do these two shades work well on you?

MIDNIGHT BLUE   EMERALD GREEN

2 Can you pull off these two hard-to-wear colors?

BLACKBERRY   BLACK

3 Is this shade not your best?

APRICOT

Interpret your results

If you answered yes to all three questions you are a Deep Winter!

If the first four shades look . . .

too warm	→	try True Winter.
too cool	→	try Deep Autumn.
too soft and deep	→	try Clear Winter.
too clear and deep	→	try Soft Summer.

Are you a True Winter?

Test out these colors

1 Do these two shades work well on you?

MEDIUM BLUE   VIVID INDIGO

2 Can you pull off these two hard-to-wear colors?

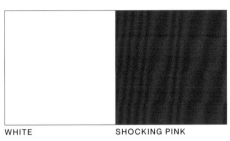

WHITE   SHOCKING PINK

3 Is this shade not your best?

SAND

Interpret your results

If you answered yes to all three questions you are a True Winter!

If the first four shades look . . .

too cool and light	→	try Deep Winter.
too cool and deep	→	try Clear Winter.
too clear and deep	→	try True Summer.

Are you a Clear Winter?

Test out these colors

1 Do these two shades work well on you?

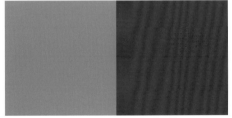

PERSIAN GREEN   FRENCH BLUE

2 Can you pull off these two hard-to-wear colors?

RUBY RED   RICH RASPBERRY

3 Is this shade not your best?

CAMEL

Interpret your results

If you answered yes to all three questions you are a Clear Winter!

If the first four shades look . . .

too warm and clear	→	try True Winter.
too cool	→	try Clear Spring.
too clear and light	→	try Deep Winter.
too clear and deep	→	try True Summer.

What to use as drapes

Ideally, your drapes will be made of some kind of fabric: clothes, sheets, towels, even your canvas weekender bag. As long as you can lift it up and hold it underneath your face, it will work!

If you cannot find a piece of fabric in the exact color you need, you can also use colored paper. In a pinch, any random object in that exact color works, as long as it is at least as wide as your face.

What's more important than the material of your drapes is their color. I'd much rather you use a plastic bag in the exact deep emerald green you need than a sweater that's really more of a deep olive. Yes, both are deep greens, but their undertone and chroma put them in completely different seasons. Of course, a 100 percent match will rarely be possible, but you should get pretty close.

The biggest mistake people make when testing out colors is a lack of attention to color accuracy. For example, I often see people applying vivid coral lipstick and then falsely concluding they must not have a warm undertone, when perhaps the problem wasn't the coral's undertone but its chroma and/or value. Your drapes should match the recommended colors in all aspects: undertone, chroma, and value.

The biggest mistake people make when testing out colors is a lack of attention to color accuracy.

Target color

Low color accuracy

Good color accuracy

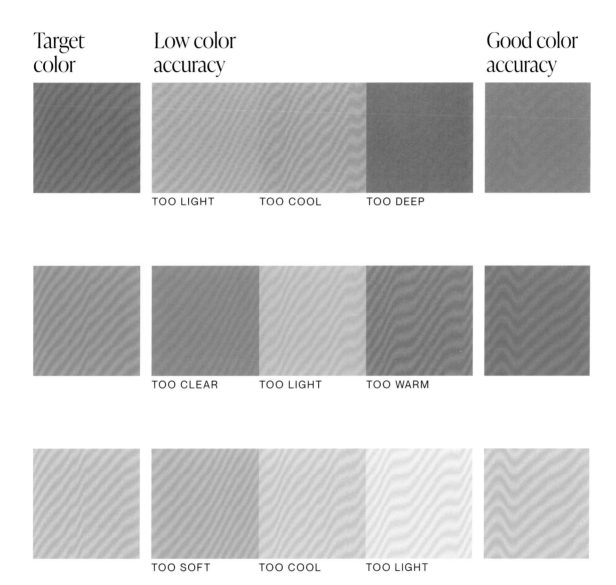

TOO LIGHT   TOO COOL   TOO DEEP

TOO CLEAR   TOO LIGHT   TOO WARM

TOO SOFT   TOO COOL   TOO LIGHT

DRAPING

157

The draping process

Just like you did for assessing your properties, I recommend you analyze the look of each drape using a photo instead of a mirror. That way you can take your time with the analysis and adjust the color balance of your photos if you need to.

All the same rules apply for your draping sessions as for your picture taking (see page 76 for a refresher). You want to be able to see your coloring as clearly and faithfully as possible, without any sort of cast from the light. Do not wear any makeup or self-tanner. If you have color-treated hair, pull it back or gel it back as much as possible. Do not use anything like a headscarf or a towel to cover your hair, as the color of these items may throw off your analysis.

Before you start your draping session, I recommend you have all of your drapes ready to go and organized by season. Hold each drape directly underneath your face. Then look into the camera and take a close-up photo (or have someone else take your photo).

After your draping session, you'll have made quite the addition to your camera roll (fifteen to thirty images). There are a few things you can do to make the reviewing process easier. For example, you could create albums or folders for each season ahead of time and drop your photos into them. Or, you could write down all three to six seasons you will be testing on scraps of paper and hold up the appropriate one when photographing a color. You could also include a gesture to indicate whether a color is supposed to be harmonious or dissonant, like a simple thumbs-up or thumbs-down. Of course, you can also label your photos afterward, if that is easier.

How to tell if a color looks harmonious

Once you have taken all your photos, it's time to assess which season's colors best harmonize with your coloring, and which dissonant colors harmonize the least. It is absolutely critical for this step that you don't let your feelings about the color itself interfere with your judgment. You might strongly prefer to keep salmon or shocking pink or mantis green out of your wardrobe, but that should not prevent you from acknowledging whether those shades harmonize with your coloring. Similarly, if you are draping a shade that you wear all the time, try your best to look at it with fresh eyes. Remember, you are not making a judgment about whether or not you'll wear these shades in the future; all drapes are simply proxies for a color season, each of which comprises many more shades. Even if you hate salmon, if it works on your coloring, you can use that valuable information to find many more flattering shades that you prefer.

As you go through your photos, ask yourself the three questions below. If you are not sure how to answer a question, or if a color just looks fine/okay/neutral, you can move on. But take note of any colors that cause a strong positive or negative response.

Do I have an immediate gut reaction?

A positive (or negative) gut reaction is often the best indicator for color harmony (or a lack thereof). Remember: Color harmony is a universal principle, and it is in our biology to respond to it favorably. If you immediately feel like a color does or does not harmonize with your coloring, that is all the information you require; you don't need to question it further.

Does this color stick out like a sore thumb?

A key indicator of color dissonance is that the color stands out. Your eyes are instantly drawn to that color, because it breaks the pattern of the rest of your coloring. If the drape is covering your neck, your head will seem to kind of float in space on the picture. A dissonant color will also look very bold and dressed up on you, regardless of what type of color it is. On the other hand, a harmonious color will look and feel effortless and natural on you. Even if it is an intense color, it will not overwhelm your features or stick out like a sore thumb.

Does this color make me look like I am wearing makeup, or like I am under the weather?

A harmonious color can have the same effect as a touch of makeup: Your skin tone appears more even; your whole complexion looks fresh and glowy. A dissonant color, on the other hand, may wash out your complexion and emphasize any shadows on your face. Sometimes a dissonant color can also emphasize certain tones in your skin. For example, if you have a cool skin tone, warm colors may make your skin appear more yellow.

Remember: The seasons on your short list *all* match your coloring to a degree, and we can expect most of their colors to look harmonious on you and not clash with your skin tone. We are looking for the gems in an already pre-vetted batch. The colors of your season will look more than just reasonably harmonious; they will feel *just right* against your coloring and give you that extra boost of radiance.

If you can identify a single season that you are instantly drawn to, congratulations—you've found your winner and can skip to Part 3 of this book to explore your color palette. But the vast majority of people get stuck between two seasons at this point. If you are one of them, the next chapter will help you out.

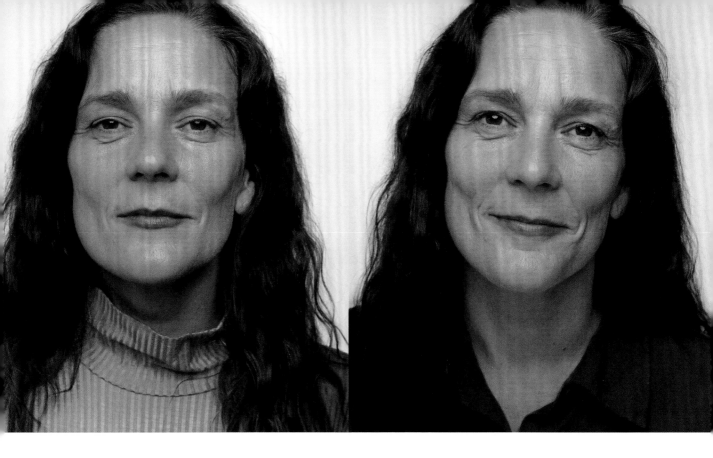

Due to her high contrast level and soft chroma, Dorte may end up with the following most likely seasons: Soft Summer, Soft Autumn, and True Autumn. Here you see her comparing a lavender (a Soft Summer shade) with a carmine red (a True Autumn shade). Dorte looks stunning in both photos, but can you see how the carmine red seems to brighten up her face, while the cool-toned lavender sticks out like a sore thumb against her warm-toned complexion? Draping both of these colors allows Dorte to conclude she is not a Summer season but rather a Soft Autumn or a True Autumn.

CLOSE CALLS

When You Can't Decide Between Two Seasons

You can confidently exclude ten seasons but struggle to decide between the last two. Perhaps you feel right in the middle of a Clear Winter and a Clear Spring? Or maybe during your draping session, the Soft Autumn colors felt just as harmonious as the True Spring ones did?

Fear not: Being stuck between two seasons is very common, and there is help! Other than sister seasons (which have a lot of overlap and are, therefore, easy to get stuck between), there are six season pairings that tend to cause some confusion for different reasons:

Clear Spring and Deep Autumn

True Spring and Soft Autumn

Light Summer and Soft Summer

Soft Summer and Deep Winter

Soft Autumn and Deep Autumn

Deep Winter and Clear Winter

In this chapter we will explore why you may be stuck in each scenario and how to use additional colors as a litmus test.

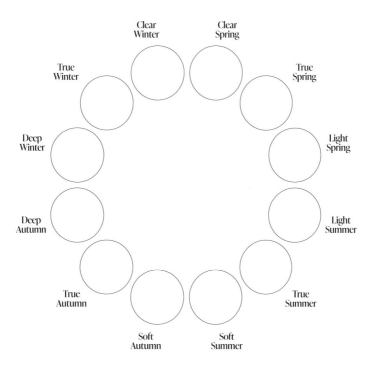

Deciding between sister seasons

There is a lot of overlap between the properties of sister types, and since you will look harmonious in both palettes, it can be hard to choose. However, there is a simple trick to make it easier: Compare your sisters' sisters!

If you struggle to decide between Light Spring and Light Summer, ask yourself whether your coloring better fits the criteria of a True Spring or True Summer—the sisters on the other side of your two contenders. Often, one of these will feel much more fitting. If your answer is True Spring, chances are your season is Light Spring. If True Summer feels more fitting, you are probably a Light Summer.

Why this works: We are amplifying the differences between the sisters so you can see them more clearly. If you are a Light Spring, it makes sense that you would identify more with True Spring than True Summer, because you can borrow colors from the True Spring palette as your sister type.

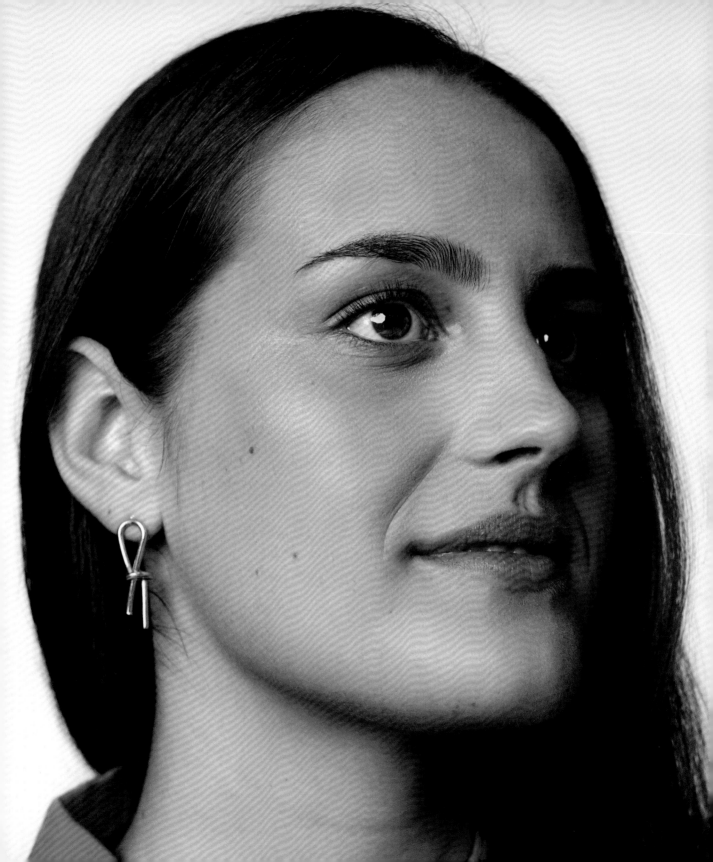

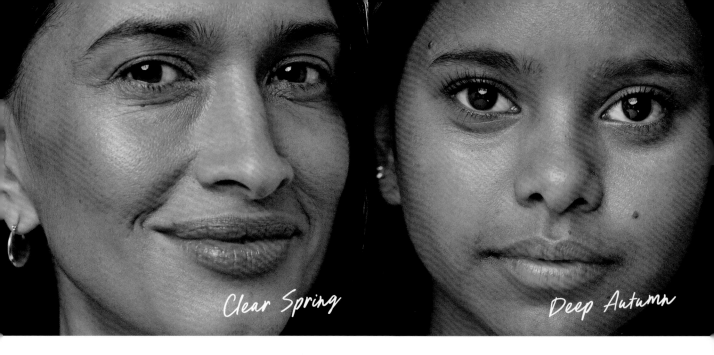

Clear Spring

Deep Autumn

Clear Spring or Deep Autumn

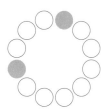

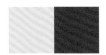

SHARED DIMENSIONS:

warm-neutral undertone, high contrast

KEY DIFFERENCE:

clear versus medium chroma

If you are deciding between these seasons it is very likely that your skin tone is light-medium or deeper. That is because Clear Springs and Deep Autumns react quite differently to colors, unless they have a light-medium or deeper skin tone, which allows Clear Springs to pull off deeper values, and can make warm-toned skin appear quite saturated, even as a medium-chroma Deep Autumn. In medium and deeper skin tones, both seasons suit rich colors of the sunset and other medium chroma, medium-deep shades. You both rock gold jewelry like no one else.

Compare a desaturated deep oak brown to a bright canary yellow. You are a Deep Autumn if the deep oak looks more harmonious than the yellow. If you like the yellow on you, and it doesn't feel like too much, you are a Clear Spring! In that case the deep oak will likely also look fine on you, but nothing to write home about. No color tends to visibly clash on Clear seasons, so the only way to confirm you are a Clear Spring (or Clear Winter) is to test out outrageously intense, even neon, shades that would overwhelm everyone else.

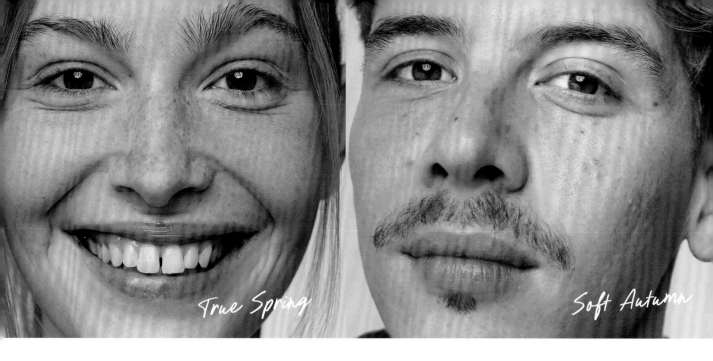

True Spring

Soft Autumn

True Spring or Soft Autumn

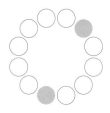

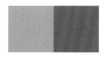

**SHARED
DIMENSIONS:**

warm or warm-
neutral undertone,
medium contrast

**KEY
DIFFERENCE:**

clear versus
soft chroma

If you are torn between these two types, it's likely that you have a deli-cate light or fair complexion and lighter features overall. Many people struggle between these two types because they feel they aren't light enough to be a True Spring or deep enough to be an Autumn season. However, Soft Autumns can have light hair and True Springs can have brown hair. The key difference between the two seasons lies in the chroma and the value of their best colors.

To differentiate between the two, you can compare a dusky gray-green to a flamingo pink. In general, pink is a good color group to rule out Autumns because the majority of shades are simply too bright or light for them (although a dusty rose works well for Soft Autumns). If the gray-green looks considerably better on you than the flamingo pink, you are a Soft Autumn and can wear deeper shades compared to the overall lightness of your coloring. Conversely, if the gray-green seems too intense or drags you down, you are a True Spring.

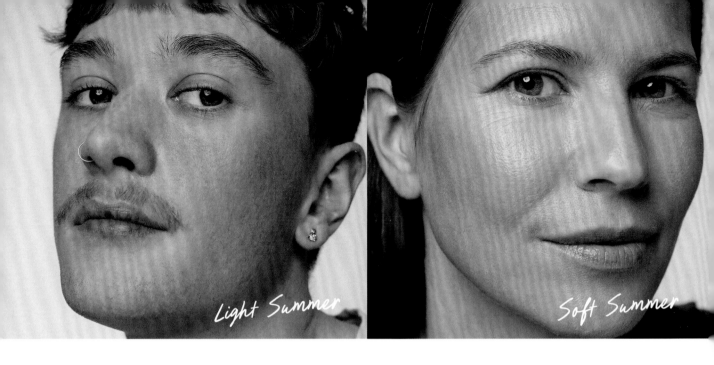

Light Summer

Soft Summer

Light Summer or Soft Summer

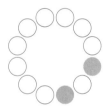

SHARED DIMENSIONS:

cool-neutral undertone, medium contrast

KEY DIFFERENCE:

medium versus soft chroma

If you are pretty sure you are some type of Summer, but your coloring isn't obviously cool, you may be stuck between these two. Both seasons will do well with medium-value, softer shades like a gentle blue or dark pink. The critical difference between them lies in the chroma of their best colors: Light Summers border on the Spring season and can handle more color intensity than Soft Summers, who, on the other hand, can pull off deeper shades.

To figure out which subtly cool Summer you are, compare a pastel lemon yellow to a dusky stone gray. Make sure the pastel yellow you are testing is not gray-based and is light but not close-to-white light. If you are a Light Summer, pastels of all kinds will harmonize with your coloring, while the deeper neutral will overpower you. The yellow may wash you out a little if you are a Soft Summer, while the deeper neutral feels just right.

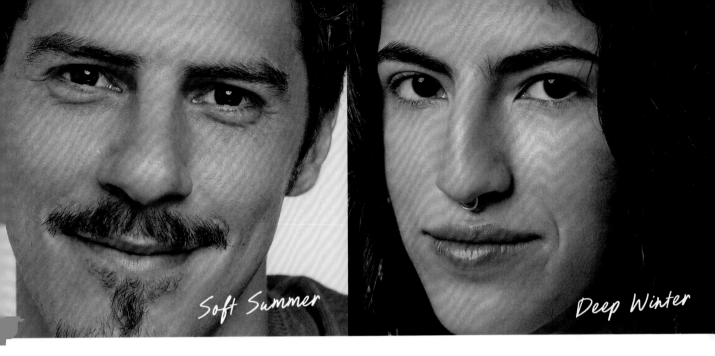

Soft Summer

Deep Winter

Soft Summer or Deep Winter

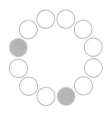

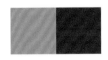

SHARED DIMENSIONS:

cool-neutral undertone, high contrast

KEY DIFFERENCE:

soft versus medium chroma

If you are deciding between Soft Summer and Deep Winter, you likely have deep features, a high contrast level, and a cool-neutral undertone. Both seasons suit deeper shades much more than light shades. Soft Summers with light-medium or deeper skin tones rock black almost as well as a Deep Winter. But when it comes to medium values, the seasons diverge considerably: Deep Winters need color intensity, and Soft Summers do better without.

First, if black looks even slightly intense on you, you are a Soft Summer. No amount of black is too overwhelming for a Deep Winter. If black looks good, compare a taupe to a blue-based shocking pink. Neither season will look amazing in either color. But as a Deep Winter, shocking pink is in your sister season's palette, so will work reasonably well, while the taupe should make you look all kinds of dull. If you are a Soft Summer, the taupe may wash you out a tad, but not as much as the pink will feel too much on all levels.

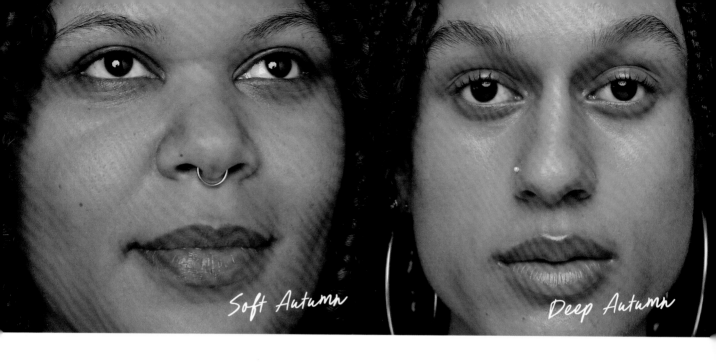

Soft Autumn

Deep Autumn

Soft Autumn or Deep Autumn

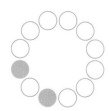

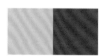

SHARED DIMENSIONS:

warm-neutral undertone, high contrast

KEY DIFFERENCE:

soft versus medium chroma

If you are torn between these two seasons, you probably have deep features, a medium to light skin tone, and balanced coloring that leans toward "neutral" in all aspects. You likely look great in all shades of browns and prefer earthy tones over pastels and bright colors.

Compare an intense pumpkin red color to a lighter, dusty rose color. Deep Autumns can pull off more intense colors compared to Soft Autumns, so if the pumpkin red feels too deep and intense against your coloring, and the dusty rose looks more harmonious (if not ideal), you are a Soft Autumn. On the other hand, if the pumpkin red works with your coloring, but the dusty rose washes you out, you are a Deep Autumn.

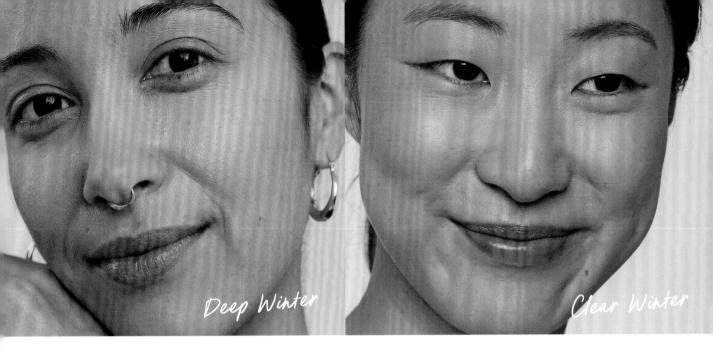

Deep Winter

Clear Winter

Deep Winter or Clear Winter

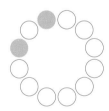

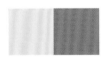

SHARED DIMENSIONS:

cool-neutral undertone, high contrast

KEY DIFFERENCE:

medium versus clear chroma

Upon first glance, Deep Winter and Clear Winter may seem similar in some ways: both have high contrast and a cool-neutral undertone. Both look great in vivid jewel tones such as jade, lapis blue, and rich magenta and can also wear the icy shades of their sister season True Winter. However, upon closer inspection, they react differently to most colors. Clear Winter requires a high level of saturation, which is why they may appear washed out in the very deep "almost black" shades that complement Deep Winter. Additionally, many bright shades that Clear Winters can pull off, such as cool pink, will intuitively look a little off on Deep Winters.

Compare a deep mustard yellow to a bright canary yellow. You are a Deep Winter if the rich mustard isn't your favorite look, but the canary yellow is far too bright and light for you. If your first reaction to the canary yellow is "not bad, actually . . ." and you don't think it looks worse than the rich mustard at all, you are a Clear Winter.

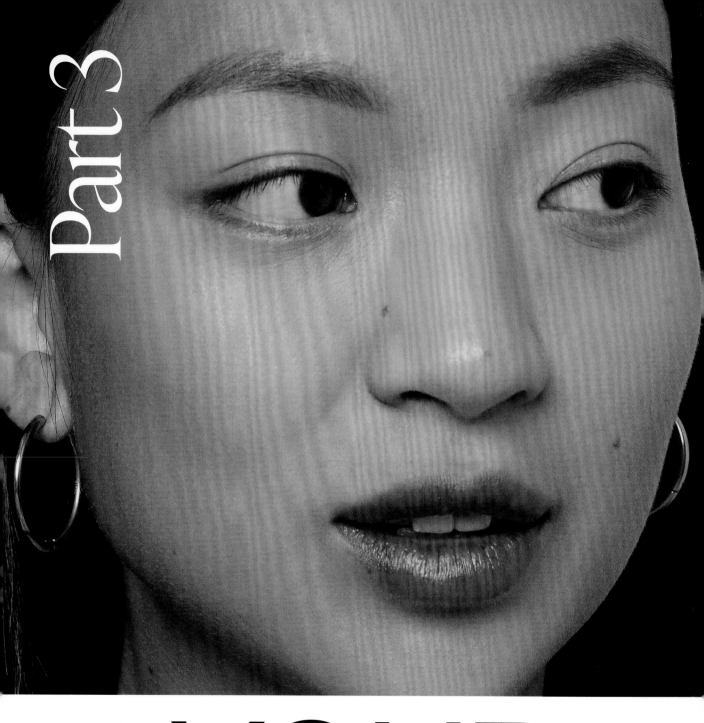

Part 3

YOUR

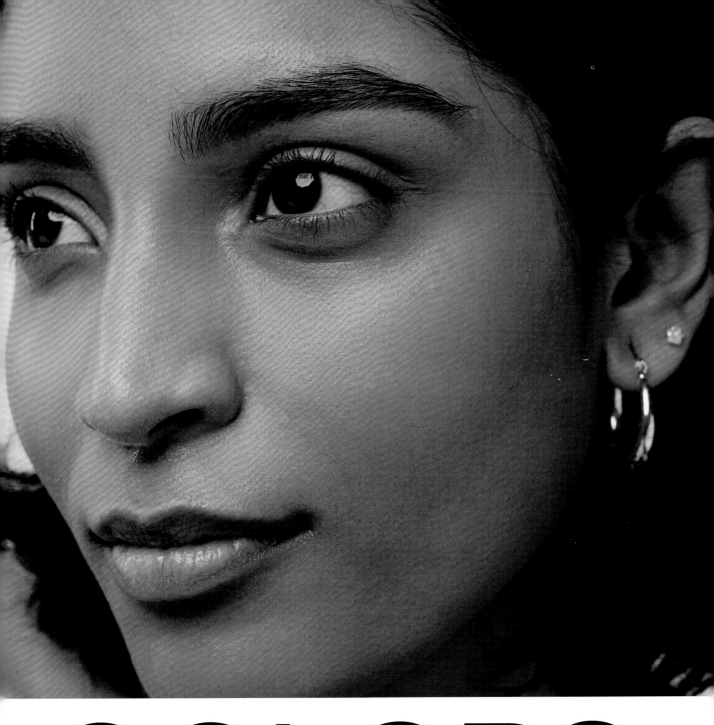

COLORS

MEET YOUR COLORS

How to Read Your Color Palette

So you've figured out your color season—congratulations! The rest of this book is dedicated to your colors: which color genres perfectly match your season, which undertones work best, and which are your "opposite colors"? You will need all of your color fluency chops, so consider flipping back to page 40 for a refresher on color genres and what determines the undertone of different hues. We will discuss hair color and makeup in the final two chapters since both depend not only on your season but also on your exact contrast level and skin tone.

The five levels of color harmony

Your season's color palette is made up of shades that perfectly echo your coloring in all three dimensions. But that doesn't mean all other colors will clash or look bad on you! Perhaps an icy blue is not a perfect match for your coloring, which is why it's not included in your palette. But if it's only a little off your ideal dimensions—for example, it has a cool undertone, while your best colors are cool-neutral—it will still look harmonious on you.

There are levels to color harmony. Some colors will be a perfect match, some will be a tad less harmonious but still work well, some will not suit you at all, and others will be neither here nor there. For a shade to look dissonant or truly clash, it needs to be pretty far removed from your coloring in all aspects.

In Part 3, we will distinguish between five levels of color harmony:

Perfect match

Your season's color palette and the colors that will truly make you shine. They perfectly honor your coloring in all dimensions and look radiant and effortless.

Harmonious

Colors that are not a perfect match, but they echo your coloring enough that they work well and look good on you. Harmonious colors are a part of your sister seasons' palettes.

Okay

Colors that are neither here nor there. They don't echo your coloring but are not quite dissonant enough to clash.

Dissonant

Colors that don't harmonize with your coloring and may overwhelm or wash out your features a little. They may also look extra bold on you, and people may notice the color before they notice your face.

Clash

Colors whose properties are (almost) the opposite of your coloring. These shades will likely visibly clash with your coloring, overwhelm your features, or wash you out.

Once you have determined your color season, we will use the levels of harmony to figure out exactly how well colors that are not a part of your palette will work with your coloring. For now, all you need to remember is that while your season's colors will be a perfect match, that does not mean all other colors will look bad. Color harmony comes in levels.

Example: If you are a Light Summer, you have a cool-neutral undertone and suit the color genre Moderates, making Picton blue a perfect match for you. Cornflower is also a Moderate but has an obviously cool undertone, so while it's not a perfect match it will still look harmonious on your coloring. A soft navy will be too deep for you, but

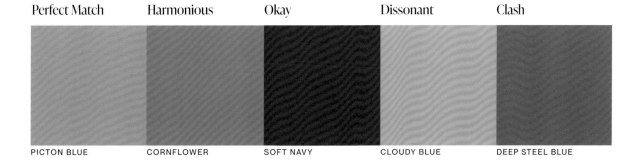

| Perfect Match | Harmonious | Okay | Dissonant | Clash |
| PICTON BLUE | CORNFLOWER | SOFT NAVY | CLOUDY BLUE | DEEP STEEL BLUE |

since its undertone and chroma (medium) match yours, it will work reasonably well. On the other hand, a cloudy blue may look dissonant since it's both too soft and a little too cool. A deep steel blue is very far removed from your coloring as a Light Summer: it's very soft, cool, and deep—and may clash with your complexion.

How aging impacts your best colors

Will different colors suit you as you get older? The short answer is yes. Our coloring changes with age, and it does so in predictable ways:

☐ Most people's undertone stays the same, although those with an obviously warm undertone (not warm-neutral) will likely prefer warm-neutral shades once their hair has gone entirely gray.

☐ Our chroma decreases due to changes in the natural luminosity and saturation of our complexion and eye color.

☐ Our contrast level goes down as our eyebrows and eyelashes become more sparse and our irises less defined and saturated. This change tends to be more pronounced in people with higher contrast levels. For example, people with a very high contrast level may come closer to a high contrast level in their sixties and seventies. Dying hair to your pre-gray shade will not restore your original contrast level.

None of these changes will bump a person to a different color season; their best colors will merely shift somewhat. For example, a True Autumn may find that the deepest shades of the True Autumn palette are less harmonious than they used to be, while the gentler Soft-Autumn-leaning shades of their palette work even better than before.

How a suntan impacts your best colors

When you tan in the sun, your existing melanocytes do their best to protect you from the sun's rays by releasing more of your unique formula of eumelanin and pheomelanin, which gives your skin its color. Some people believe that a tan allows them to pull off a larger variety of colors than usual. These individuals are often light-skinned Summers with a cool, low-chroma skin tone whose complexion becomes more saturated and warm due to an increase in pheomelanin. As a result, these individuals can indeed pull off warmer and clearer colors when tanned.

If your skin tone is medium or deeper, a suntan will also increase your skin's chroma, but it won't make it any warmer. That is because your undertone is likely due to the dominant hue of pheomelanin, rather than a lack of pheomelanin. Since the same type of pheomelanin gets released when you tan, the hue of your skin won't change. A suntan will not affect your contrast level.

In your season's section, you'll learn more about how both aging and a suntan may affect your best colors.

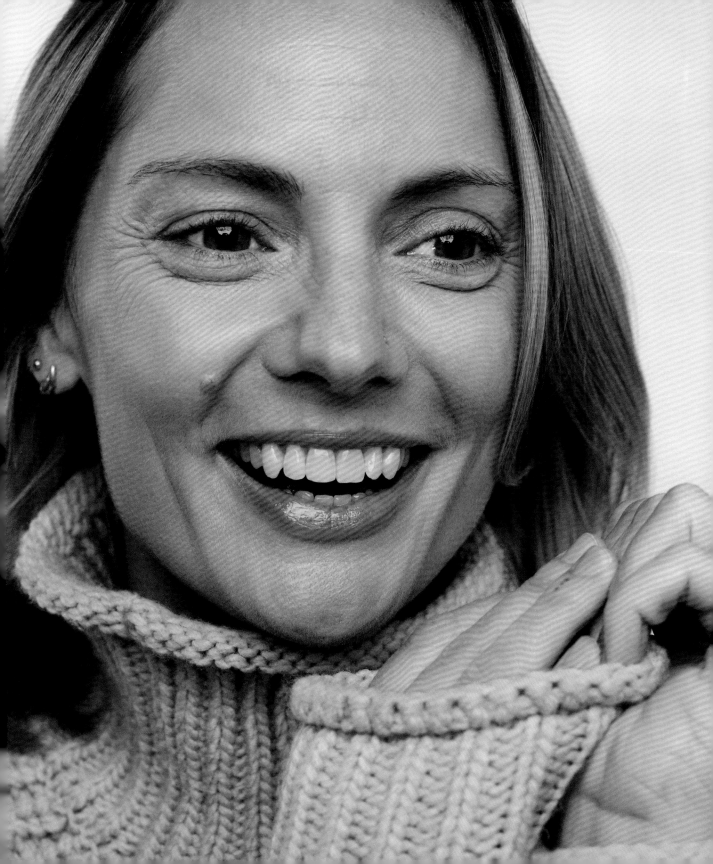

CLEAR SPRING

Color essence Vibrant and luminous

Best colors Warm-neutral Brights, Vivids, and Jewel Tones

The Clear Spring coloring combines the warm luminosity of the Spring seasons with the higher contrast intensity of the Winter seasons. Your coloring is naturally vibrant, rich, and luminous. Unlike other Spring seasons, your coloring comes with a good amount of built-in intensity, which allows you to pull off the most vibrant shades out there.

Clear Springs are often mistyped as Deep Autumns or even Winters due to their natural intensity and higher contrast level and because many people associate the Spring season with lighter features. But while Clear Springs can have lighter hair and eyes, most have a deeper coloring.

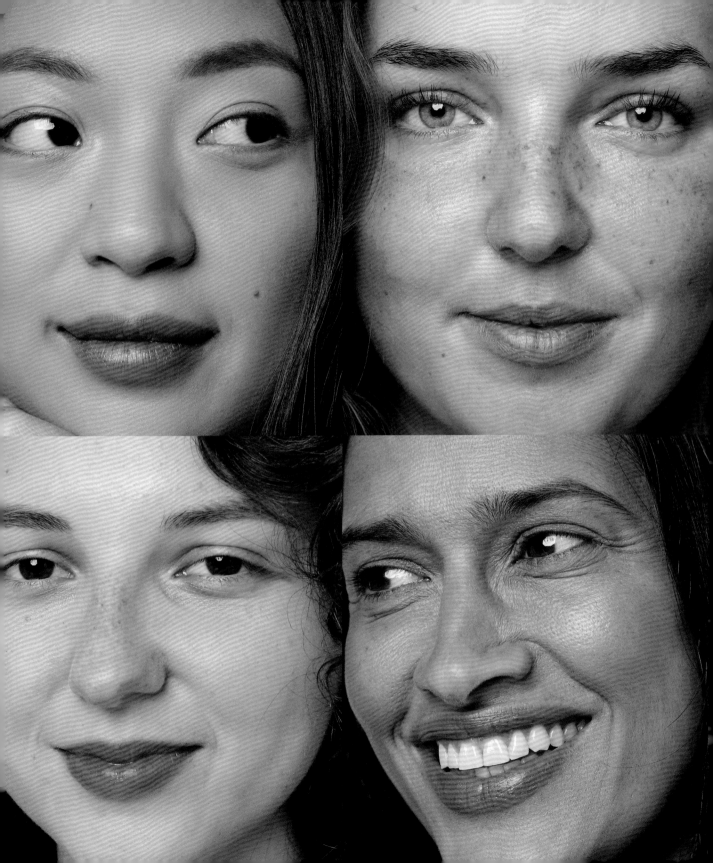

Your best colors

You need saturation above all. All three clear-chroma color genres were made for you: Brights, Vivids, and Jewel Tones. The medium-chroma genres—Pastels, Moderates, and Rich Shades—are too soft. As a warm-neutral season, your best colors echo that undertone across all seasons.

Let's look at some shades that are a perfect match for Clear Springs:

Warm-neutral Brights

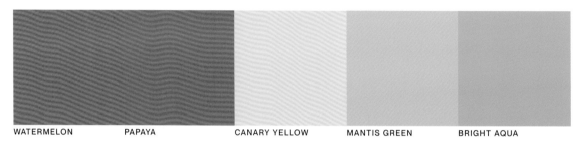

WATERMELON   PAPAYA   CANARY YELLOW   MANTIS GREEN   BRIGHT AQUA

Warm-neutral Vivids

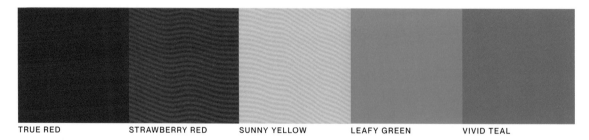

TRUE RED   STRAWBERRY RED   SUNNY YELLOW   LEAFY GREEN   VIVID TEAL

Warm-neutral Jewel Tones (*light-medium or deeper skin tones*)

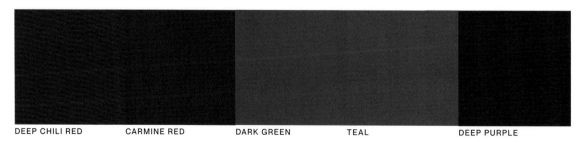

DEEP CHILI RED   CARMINE RED   DARK GREEN   TEAL   DEEP PURPLE

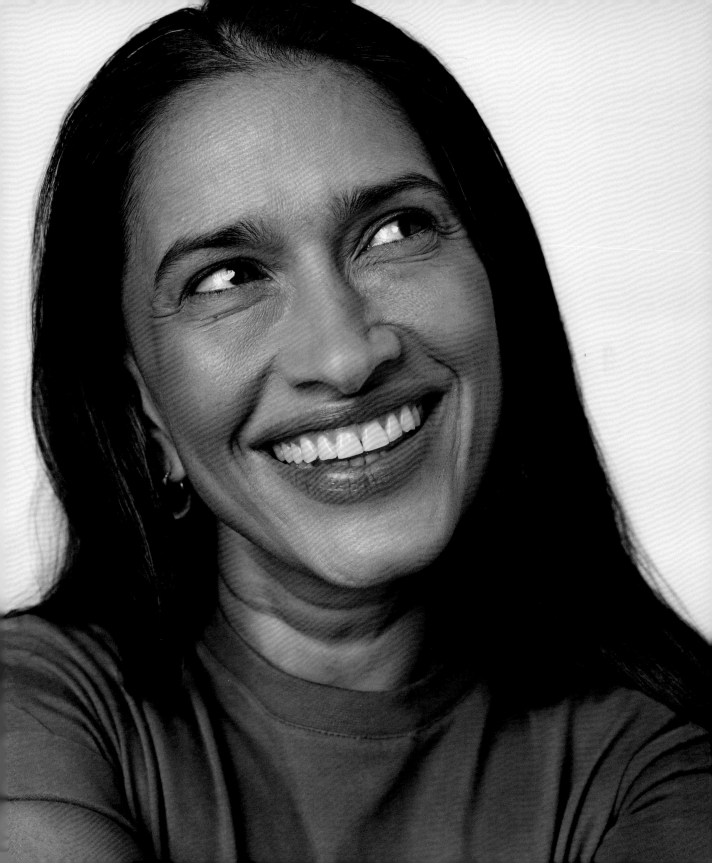

Levels of harmony

Pssst . . . don't tell the others: As a Clear Spring you are the closest there is to "looks good in everything." Due to your natural radiance, higher intensity, and close-to-neutral undertone, no shade will visibly clash with your coloring. But you'll truly come to life in warm-neutral Brights, Vivids, and Jewel Tones.

Moderates are not a perfect match, but they're still a good choice for Clear Springs, especially in a warm-neutral undertone.

Here is an overview of how well different undertones and color genres work on Clear Springs. Ratings for color genres are based on shades that match your best undertone (warm-neutral). Shades in other undertones will be less harmonious.

	Color genre	Undertone
PERFECT MATCH	Brights Vivids Jewel Tones *(light-medium or deeper skin tones)*	Warm-neutral
HARMONIOUS	Moderates	Warm Cool-neutral
OKAY	Pastels Rich Shades Jewel Tones *(light and fair skin tones)*	Cool
DISSONANT	Dusky Shades	
CLASH	Dimmed Tones Pale Tones	

Your "opposite" colors

Cool-toned Dimmed Tones and Pale Tones are your least harmonious colors. They don't echo any aspect of your coloring and may clash with your complexion. Here are some examples:

Cool Dimmed Tones

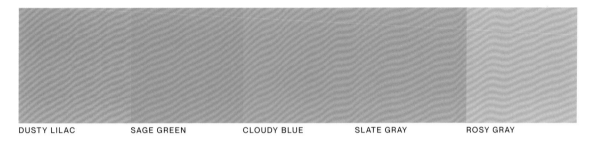

DUSTY LILAC   SAGE GREEN   CLOUDY BLUE   SLATE GRAY   ROSY GRAY

Cool Pale Tones

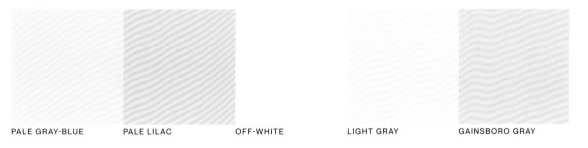

PALE GRAY-BLUE   PALE LILAC   OFF-WHITE   LIGHT GRAY   GAINSBORO GRAY

How aging may affect your best colors

Like all seasons, Clear Springs lose some of their chroma and contrast with age. This means that the Brights and Jewel Tones in your palette may start to look slightly less harmonious, while Moderates and Pastels may become more harmonious. The undertone of your best colors will remain stable throughout your life.

How a suntan may affect your best colors

If your skin tone is fair or light, a strong suntan will warm up your complexion. As a result, you'll likely do just as well with warm hues as with warm-neutral ones. Regardless of your skin tone, a strong suntan will also increase your chroma somewhat, allowing you to pull off fluorescent, neon colors.

Best colors by hue

The Clear Spring palette features mostly warm-neutral shades that perfectly echo your softly golden coloring. For added variety, it also includes a few obviously warm shades and even cool-neutral colors, all of which Clear Springs tend to do well with. The only undertone you won't find in your palette is cool hues (including black, white, and all other grayscale shades).

This section will look at your full color palette, broken down by hue. Note that we will cover hair colors, makeup, and jewelry in later chapters.

Red and pink

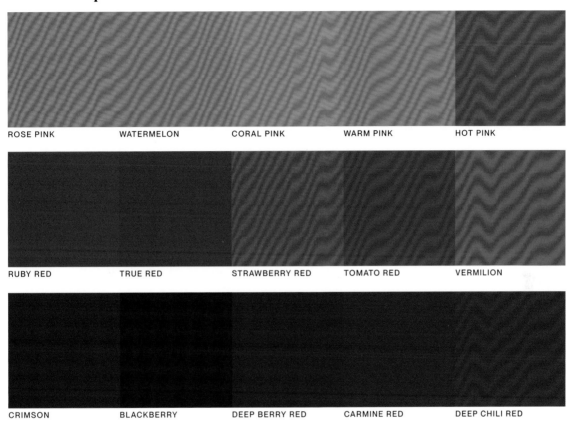

ROSE PINK   WATERMELON   CORAL PINK   WARM PINK   HOT PINK

RUBY RED   TRUE RED   STRAWBERRY RED   TOMATO RED   VERMILION

CRIMSON   BLACKBERRY   DEEP BERRY RED   CARMINE RED   DEEP CHILI RED

Orange and yellow

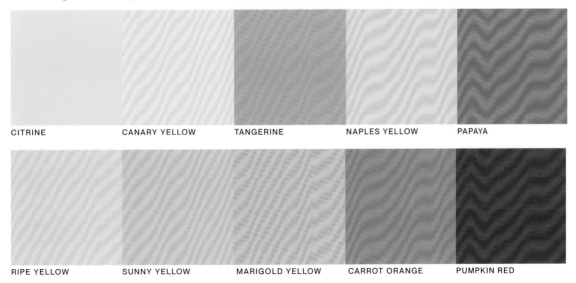

CITRINE   CANARY YELLOW   TANGERINE   NAPLES YELLOW   PAPAYA

RIPE YELLOW   SUNNY YELLOW   MARIGOLD YELLOW   CARROT ORANGE   PUMPKIN RED

Green

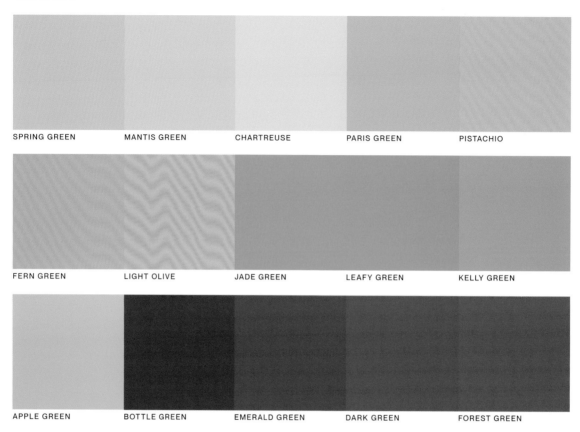

SPRING GREEN   MANTIS GREEN   CHARTREUSE   PARIS GREEN   PISTACHIO

FERN GREEN   LIGHT OLIVE   JADE GREEN   LEAFY GREEN   KELLY GREEN

APPLE GREEN   BOTTLE GREEN   EMERALD GREEN   DARK GREEN   FOREST GREEN

Cyan and blue

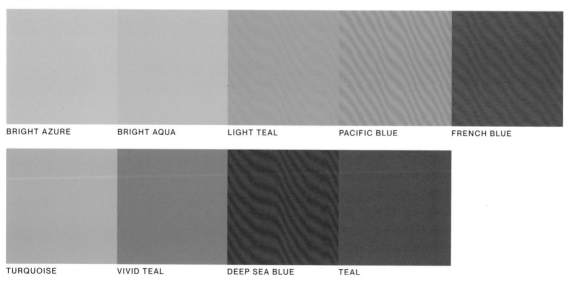

BRIGHT AZURE   BRIGHT AQUA   LIGHT TEAL   PACIFIC BLUE   FRENCH BLUE

TURQUOISE   VIVID TEAL   DEEP SEA BLUE   TEAL

Violet

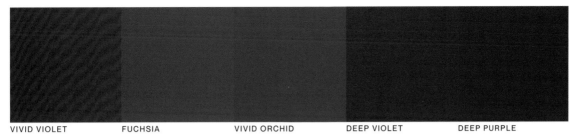

VIVID VIOLET FUCHSIA VIVID ORCHID DEEP VIOLET DEEP PURPLE

Neutrals

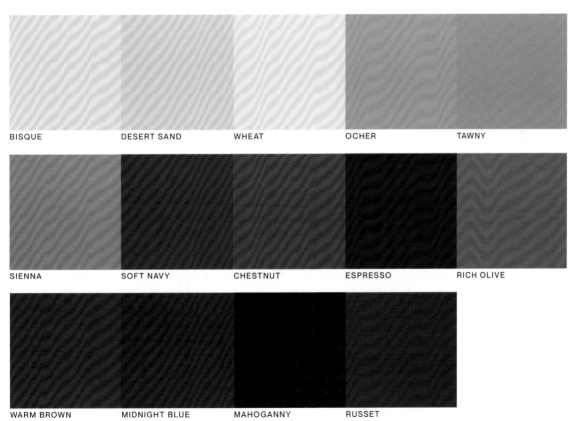

BISQUE DESERT SAND WHEAT OCHER TAWNY

SIENNA SOFT NAVY CHESTNUT ESPRESSO RICH OLIVE

WARM BROWN MIDNIGHT BLUE MAHOGANNY RUSSET

TRUE SPRING

Color essence Warm and luminous
Best colors Warm Brights and Moderates

True Springs are the archetypal Spring types: warm, clear, and radiant. Your coloring comes preinstalled with a ton of luminosity, and your best colors are equally bright and sunny. Although some True Springs have lighter features, brown eyes and hair are typical in medium to deeper skin tones.

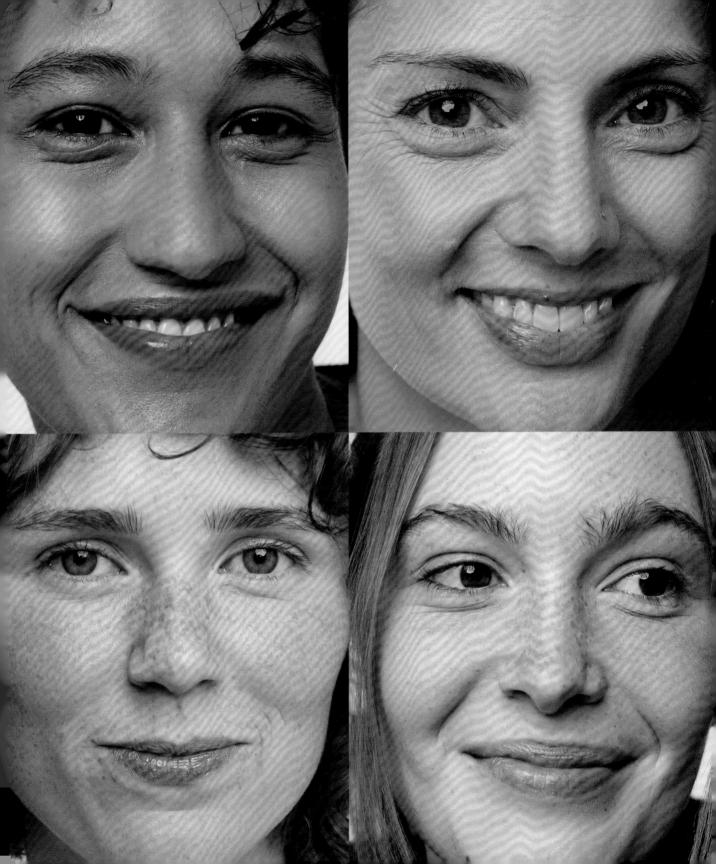

Your best colors

True Spring colors are suited by what is sometimes called the Crayola palette of the seasons: saturated, bright hues, with not a muddy, faded shade in sight. True Springs are the only season with clear chroma but without a high contrast level. That means you require color intensity but cannot handle a lot of depth. Your best color genres are Brights and Moderates. If your skin tone is light-medium or deeper, you will also look great in Jewel Tones. Across all color genres, warm shades work best for your warm undertone. Here is a selection of shades that perfectly echo your coloring:

Warm Brights

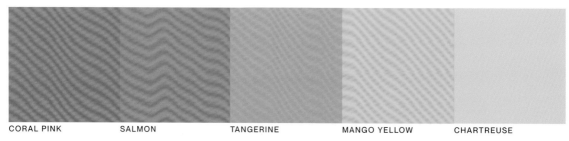

| CORAL PINK | SALMON | TANGERINE | MANGO YELLOW | CHARTREUSE |

Warm Moderates

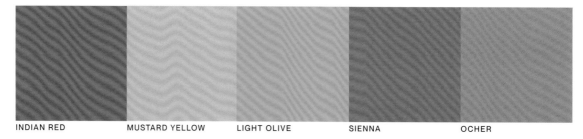

| INDIAN RED | MUSTARD YELLOW | LIGHT OLIVE | SIENNA | OCHER |

Warm Jewel Tones (*light-medium or deeper skin tones*)

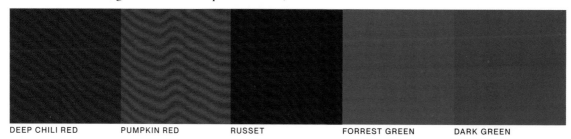

| DEEP CHILI RED | PUMPKIN RED | RUSSET | FORREST GREEN | DARK GREEN |

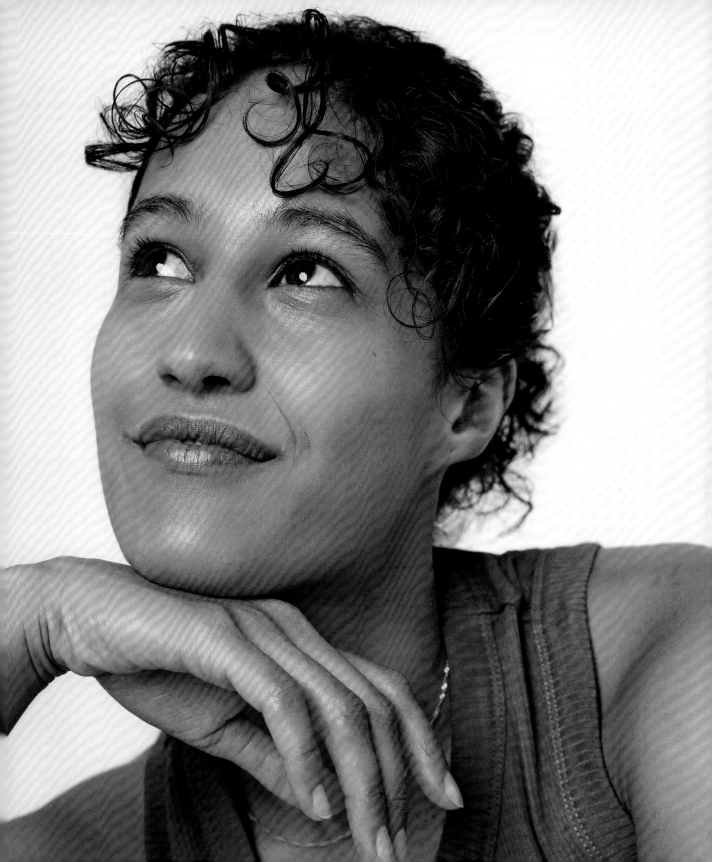

Levels of harmony

True Springs shine in Brights and Moderates with a warm undertone. But what about other types of colors? Although your undertone is pronounced, you have an advantage over obviously cool seasons, whose complexions tend to clash with any amount of visible warmth. Warm seasons look better in warm shades than cool ones, but they can tolerate cool colors just fine. A cool-neutral shade like a rose pink won't look dissonant on a True Spring, the way a papaya hue would on a True Summer.

When it comes to color genres, Vivids are almost as good of a match as Brights and Moderates. Contrary to popular belief, Pastels are not an ideal choice for True Springs, as they are often too light to

	Color genre	Undertone
PERFECT MATCH	Brights Moderates Jewel Tones *(light-medium or deeper skin tones)*	Warm
HARMONIOUS	Vivids Pastels	Warm-neutral
OKAY	Jewel Tones *(fair or light skin tones)* Rich Shades Pale Tones	Cool-neutral
DISSONANT	Dimmed Tones	Cool
CLASH	Dusky Shades	

contain enough saturation. Although in a warm undertone, they will still look harmonious. However, Pale Tones tend to wash out the Spring complexion.

On the previous page is an overview of how well different undertones and color genres work on True Springs. Ratings for color genres are based on shades that match your best undertone (warm). Shades in other undertones will be less harmonious.

Your "opposite" colors

Cool-toned Dusky Shades are your least harmonious colors. They don't echo any aspect of your coloring and may clash with your complexion. Here are some examples of cool Dusky Shades:

Cool Dusky Shades

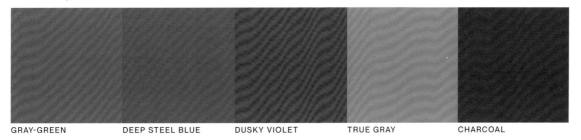

| GRAY-GREEN | DEEP STEEL BLUE | DUSKY VIOLET | TRUE GRAY | CHARCOAL |

How aging may affect your best colors

Like all seasons, True Springs lose some of their chroma and contrast with age. This means that the Brights in your palette may start to look slightly less harmonious, while Pastels may become more harmonious. As a warm season, your undertone may also become slightly less pronounced with age, and you may gravitate to warm-neutral colors.

How a suntan may affect your best colors

If your skin tone is fair or light, a strong suntan will warm up your complexion, allowing you to truly rock the warmest shades of your palette. Regardless of your skin tone, a strong suntan will also slightly increase your chroma, making Vivids one of your best color genres.

Best colors by hue

This section will look at your full color palette, broken down by hue. Note that we will cover hair colors, makeup, and jewelry in later chapters! Jewel Tones are a perfect match for True Springs with a light-medium or deeper skin tone only and are marked with an asterisk.

Red and pink

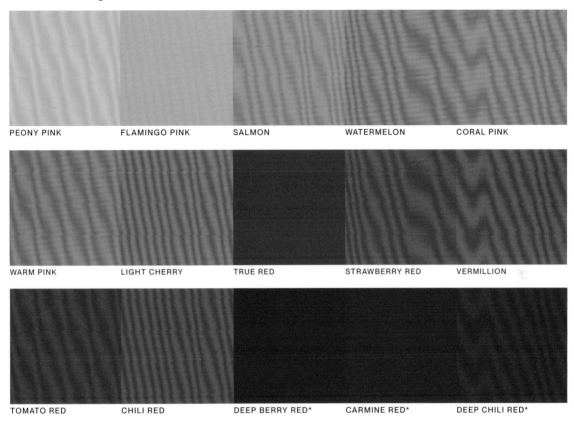

PEONY PINK	FLAMINGO PINK	SALMON	WATERMELON	CORAL PINK
WARM PINK	LIGHT CHERRY	TRUE RED	STRAWBERRY RED	VERMILLION
TOMATO RED	CHILI RED	DEEP BERRY RED*	CARMINE RED*	DEEP CHILI RED*

Orange and yellow

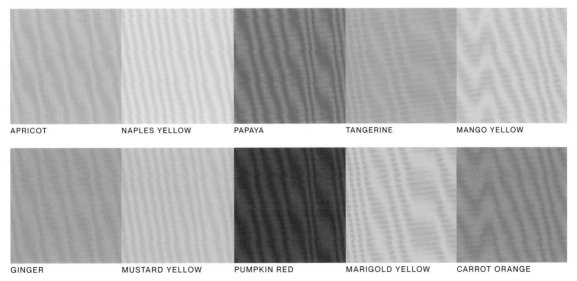

APRICOT	NAPLES YELLOW	PAPAYA	TANGERINE	MANGO YELLOW
GINGER	MUSTARD YELLOW	PUMPKIN RED	MARIGOLD YELLOW	CARROT ORANGE

Green

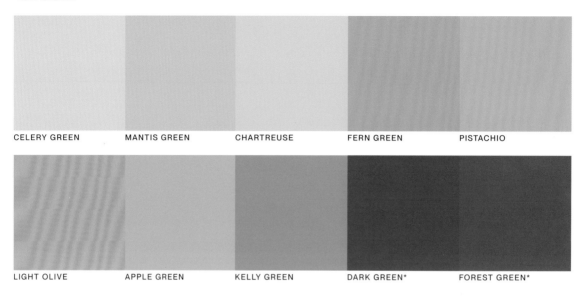

CELERY GREEN   MANTIS GREEN   CHARTREUSE   FERN GREEN   PISTACHIO

LIGHT OLIVE   APPLE GREEN   KELLY GREEN   DARK GREEN*   FOREST GREEN*

Cyan and blue

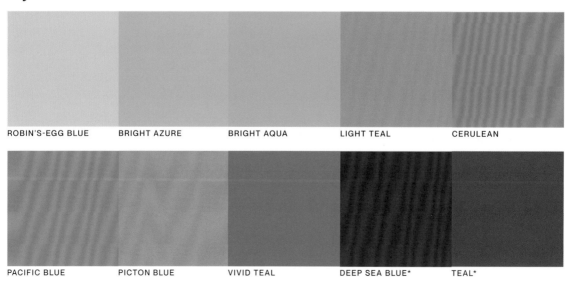

ROBIN'S-EGG BLUE   BRIGHT AZURE   BRIGHT AQUA   LIGHT TEAL   CERULEAN

PACIFIC BLUE   PICTON BLUE   VIVID TEAL   DEEP SEA BLUE*   TEAL*

Neutrals

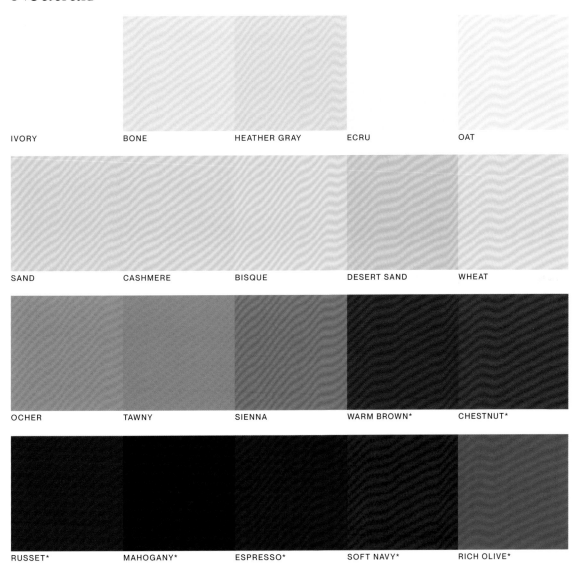

IVORY   BONE   HEATHER GRAY   ECRU   OAT

SAND   CASHMERE   BISQUE   DESERT SAND   WHEAT

OCHER   TAWNY   SIENNA   WARM BROWN*   CHESTNUT*

RUSSET*   MAHOGANY*   ESPRESSO*   SOFT NAVY*   RICH OLIVE*

Note: Since your best color genres do not offer many neutral shades, the selection here also includes
Rich Shades and Pale Tones.

LIGHT SPRING

Color essence Delicate and radiant
Best colors Warm-neutral Pastels
and Moderates

Like all Spring seasons, your coloring is naturally luminous and radiant, and you shine in warm, saturated colors. But you also have one foot in the Summer season, which makes you considerably softer and more delicate than the rest of your Spring family.

Contrary to popular belief, not all Light Springs have particularly light features. While many natural blonds and redheads are a part of this season, medium skin tones and brown hair are just as common. But overall, Light Spring is one of the less diverse seasons.

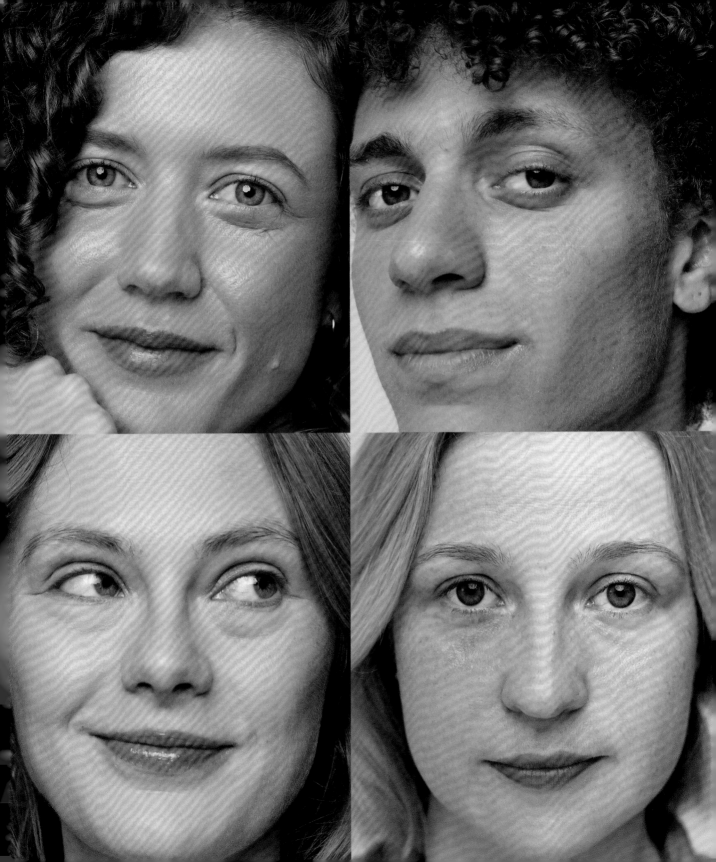

Your best colors

The Light Spring palette is a lightweight, softer version of the warm Crayola hues of Spring. As a low- to medium-contrast season, many color genres are too deep or vivid for your coloring. At the same time, you need a certain level of saturation. Two color genres tick your boxes: Pastels and Moderates. You will also look great in Rich Shades if your skin tone is light-medium or deeper. Across all color genres, warm-neutral shades best echo your undertone. Here are some examples of shades that complement Light Springs perfectly:

Warm-neutral Pastels

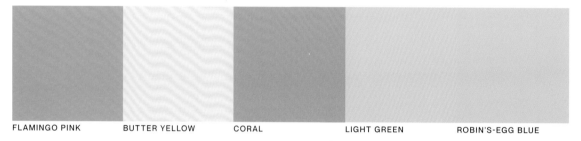

FLAMINGO PINK   BUTTER YELLOW   CORAL   LIGHT GREEN   ROBIN'S-EGG BLUE

Warm-neutral Moderates

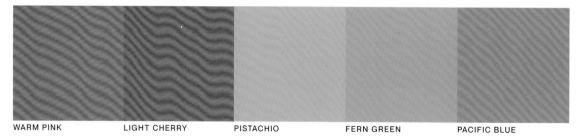

WARM PINK   LIGHT CHERRY   PISTACHIO   FERN GREEN   PACIFIC BLUE

Warm-neutral Rich Shades (*light-medium or deeper skin tones*)

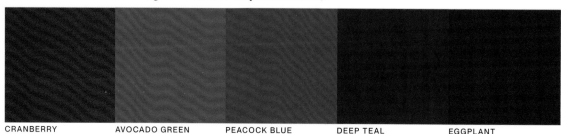

CRANBERRY   AVOCADO GREEN   PEACOCK BLUE   DEEP TEAL   EGGPLANT

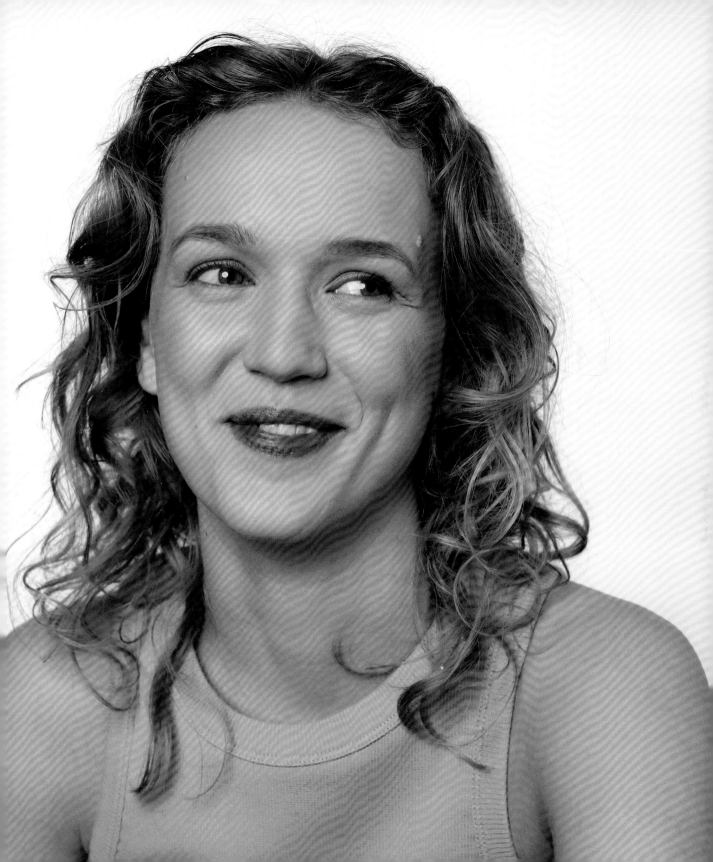

Levels of harmony

As a Light Spring, your best colors are warm-neutral Pastels and Moderates, but that doesn't mean all other types of colors look bad! While warm-neutral shades optimally echo your own undertone, warm shades will also harmonize with your coloring, and even cool-neutral shades will look fine. Only obviously cool shades may clash with your complexion, and drag down your natural radiance.

Brights can appear a little intense on your coloring, but they can still look good as long as they honor your warm-neutral undertone. Pale Tones can also look reasonably harmonious despite being on the softer side of ideal for you.

	Color genre	Undertone
PERFECT MATCH	Pastels Moderates Rich Shades (*light-medium or deeper skin tones*)	Warm-neutral
HARMONIOUS	Brights Pale Tones	Warm Cool-neutral
OKAY	Vivids Rich Shades (*fair or light skin tones*)	Cool
DISSONANT	Dimmed Tones Jewel Tones	
CLASH	Dusky Shades	

To the left is an overview of how well different undertones and color genres work on Light Springs. Ratings for color genres are based on shades that match your best undertone (warm-neutral)—shades in other undertones will be less harmonious.

Your "opposite" colors

Cool-toned Dusky Shades are your least harmonious colors. They don't echo any aspect of your coloring, and may clash with your complexion. Here are some examples of cool Dusky Shades:

Cool Dusky Shades

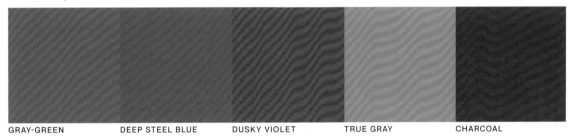

GRAY-GREEN   DEEP STEEL BLUE   DUSKY VIOLET   TRUE GRAY   CHARCOAL

How aging may affect your best colors

Like all seasons, Light Springs lose some of their chroma and contrast with age. This means that Brights and any deeper shades may start to look slightly less harmonious, while Pale Tones may become more harmonious. The undertone of your best colors will remain stable throughout your life.

How a suntan may affect your best colors

If your skin tone is fair or light, a strong suntan will warm up your complexion. As a result, you'll likely do just as well with warm hues as with warm-neutral ones. Regardless of your skin tone, a strong suntan will also increase your chroma somewhat, making Brights a perfect match for you.

Best colors by hue

In this section, we will take a look at your full color palette, broken down by hue. Note that we will cover hair colors, makeup, and jewelry in later chapters! Rich Shades are a perfect match for Light Springs with a light-medium or deeper skin tone only and are marked with an asterisk.

Red and pink

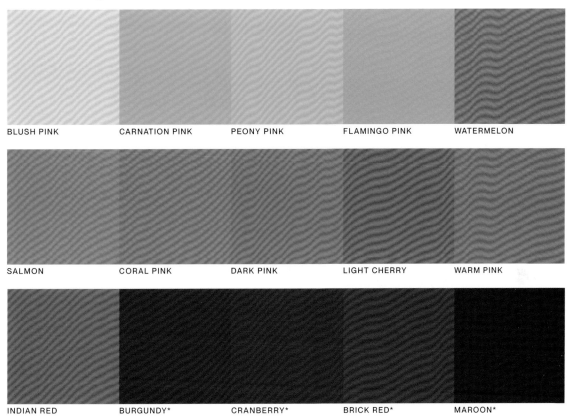

BLUSH PINK	CARNATION PINK	PEONY PINK	FLAMINGO PINK	WATERMELON
SALMON	CORAL PINK	DARK PINK	LIGHT CHERRY	WARM PINK
INDIAN RED	BURGUNDY*	CRANBERRY*	BRICK RED*	MAROON*

Orange and yellow

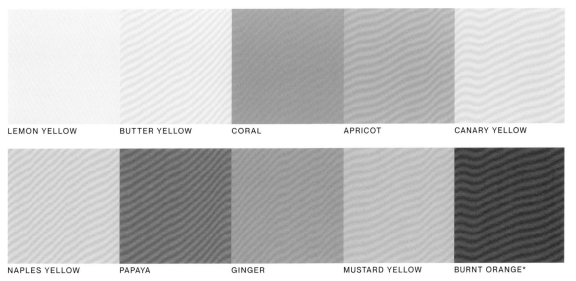

| LEMON YELLOW | BUTTER YELLOW | CORAL | APRICOT | CANARY YELLOW |
| NAPLES YELLOW | PAPAYA | GINGER | MUSTARD YELLOW | BURNT ORANGE* |

Green

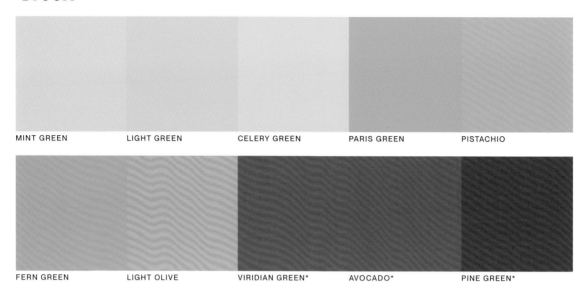

MINT GREEN   LIGHT GREEN   CELERY GREEN   PARIS GREEN   PISTACHIO

FERN GREEN   LIGHT OLIVE   VIRIDIAN GREEN*   AVOCADO*   PINE GREEN*

Cyan and blue

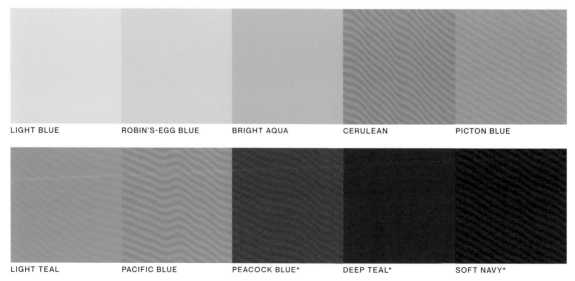

LIGHT BLUE   ROBIN'S-EGG BLUE   BRIGHT AQUA   CERULEAN   PICTON BLUE

LIGHT TEAL   PACIFIC BLUE   PEACOCK BLUE*   DEEP TEAL*   SOFT NAVY*

Violet

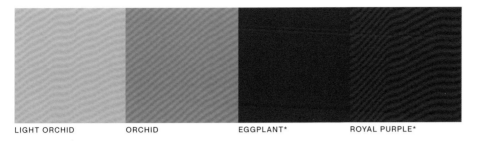

LIGHT ORCHID   ORCHID   EGGPLANT*   ROYAL PURPLE*

Neutrals

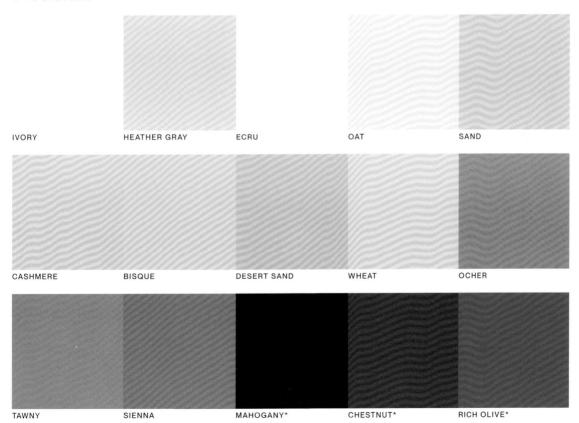

IVORY   HEATHER GRAY   ECRU   OAT   SAND

CASHMERE   BISQUE   DESERT SAND   WHEAT   OCHER

TAWNY   SIENNA   MAHOGANY*   CHESTNUT*   RICH OLIVE*

LIGHT SUMMER

Color essence Delicate and lightweight
Best colors Cool-neutral Pastels and Moderates

Light Summers toe the line between the bright and radiant Spring season and the gentle, serene Summer season. Your coloring is delicate and airy but also characteristically balanced.

While some Light Summers have very light features, most do not. If you are a part of this majority, you may have struggled to determine your season because your coloring appears "medium," with no extremes in either color dimension. Your chroma is somewhere between soft and clear, and your undertone may appear neither warm nor particularly cool. This balance is a feature of the Light Summer season, and it means you can pull off a broad range of hues, color genres, hair colors, and even jewelry shades.

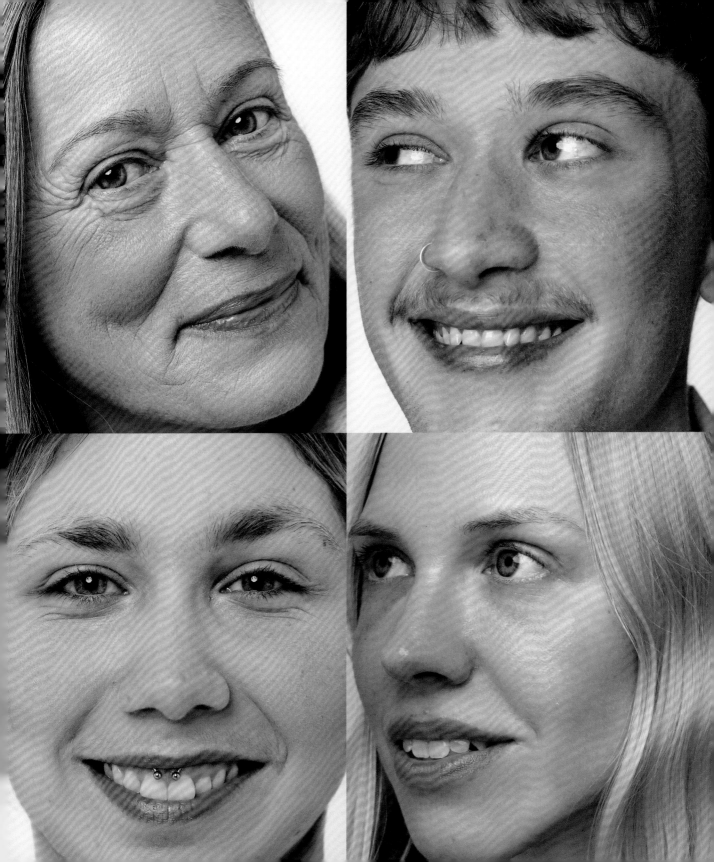

Your best colors

The Light Summer palette is fresh, lightweight, and balanced. Despite being a Summer season, you need a certain saturation level and light to medium values. Your best color genres are Pastels and Moderates. Rich Shades will also work well if your skin tone is light-medium or deeper.

Across all color genres, cool-neutral shades are a perfect match for your undertone. This is what your best color genres look like in cool-neutral versions:

Cool-neutral Pastels

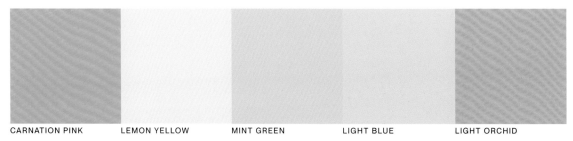

| CARNATION PINK | LEMON YELLOW | MINT GREEN | LIGHT BLUE | LIGHT ORCHID |

Cool-neutral Moderates

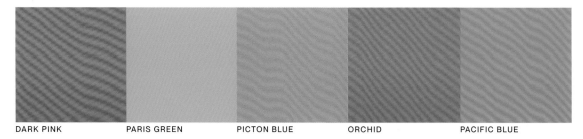

| DARK PINK | PARIS GREEN | PICTON BLUE | ORCHID | PACIFIC BLUE |

Cool-neutral Rich Shades (*light-medium or deeper skin tones*)

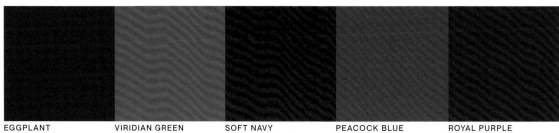

| EGGPLANT | VIRIDIAN GREEN | SOFT NAVY | PEACOCK BLUE | ROYAL PURPLE |

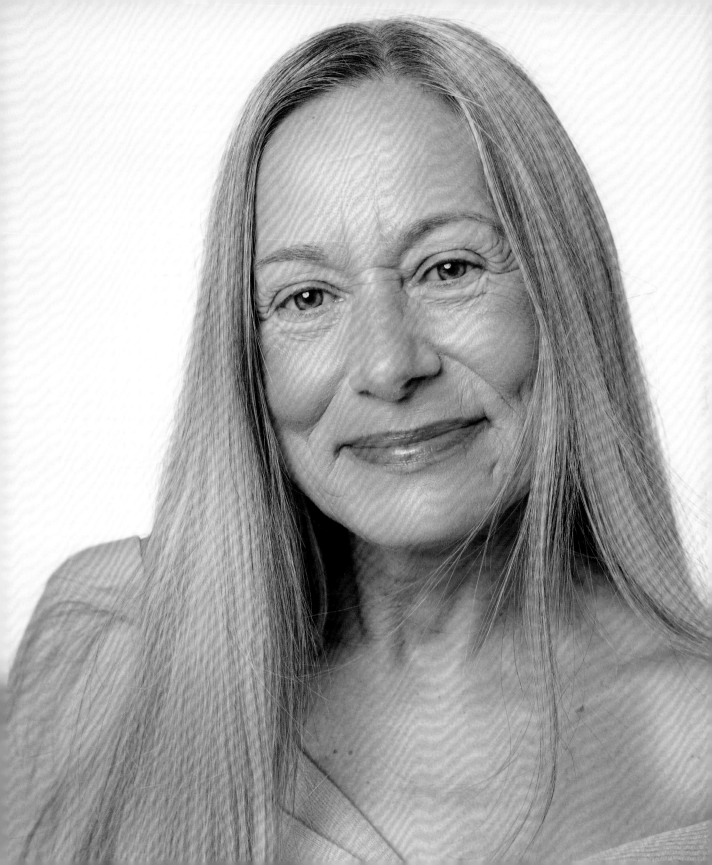

Levels of harmony

You already know that cool-neutral Pastels and Moderates look great on Light Summers. But what about other types of colors?

Although not a perfect match, Pale Tones will look good on you, especially if you choose cool-neutral versions. Brights can appear a little stark against your complexion but still work.

When it comes to undertone, you shine the most in cool-neutral colors, but you can also wear shades with a cool undertone, especially from your best color genres. Cool seasons have a harder time with warm colors than vice versa. So even though your undertone is

	Color genre	Undertone
PERFECT MATCH	Pastels Moderates Rich Shades (*light-medium or deeper skin tones*)	Cool-neutral
HARMONIOUS	Brights Pale Tones	Cool
OKAY	Vivids Rich Shades (*fair or light skin tones*)	Warm-neutral
DISSONANT	Dimmed Tones Jewel Tones	Warm
CLASH	Dusky Shades	

barely cool, warm-neutral shades will only look okay (not harmonious). Warm shades may clash with your skin tone.

To the left is an overview of how well different undertones and color genres work on Light Summers. Ratings for color genres are based on shades that match your best undertone (cool-neutral). Shades in other undertones will be less harmonious.

Your "opposite" colors

Warm Dusky Shades are your least harmonious colors. They don't echo any aspect of your coloring, and may clash with your complexion. Here are some examples:

Warm Dusky Shades

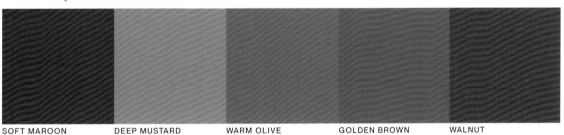

| SOFT MAROON | DEEP MUSTARD | WARM OLIVE | GOLDEN BROWN | WALNUT |

How aging may affect your best colors

Like all seasons, Light Summers lose some of their chroma and contrast with age. This means that the Brights in your palette may start to look slightly less harmonious, while Pale Tones may become more harmonious. The undertone of your best colors will remain stable throughout your life.

How a suntan may affect your best colors

If your skin tone is fair or light, a strong suntan will warm up your complexion. As a result, warm-neutral hues will likely look harmonious instead of okay. Regardless of your skin tone, a strong suntan will also increase your chroma somewhat, making Brights a perfect match for you.

Best colors by hue

Due to your balanced overall coloring, your best colors feature all eight hue families and a good selection of neutrals.

This section will look at your full color palette, broken down by hue. Note that we will cover hair colors, makeup, and jewelry in later chapters! Rich Shades are a perfect match for Light Summers with a light-medium or deeper skin tone only and are marked with an asterisk.

Red and pink

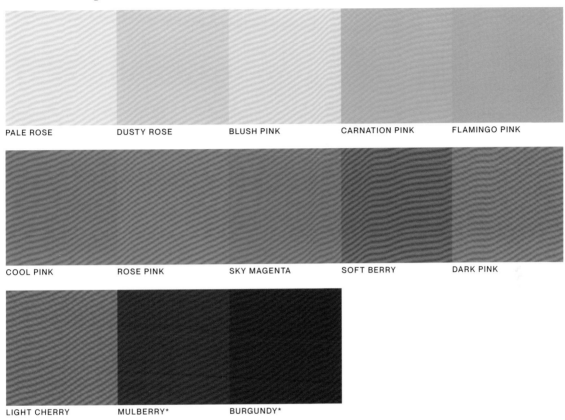

PALE ROSE

DUSTY ROSE

BLUSH PINK

CARNATION PINK

FLAMINGO PINK

COOL PINK

ROSE PINK

SKY MAGENTA

SOFT BERRY

DARK PINK

LIGHT CHERRY

MULBERRY*

BURGUNDY*

Orange and yellow

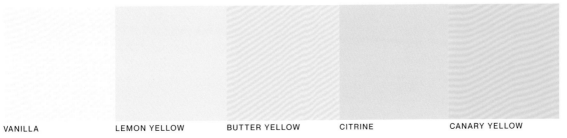

VANILLA

LEMON YELLOW

BUTTER YELLOW

CITRINE

CANARY YELLOW

Green

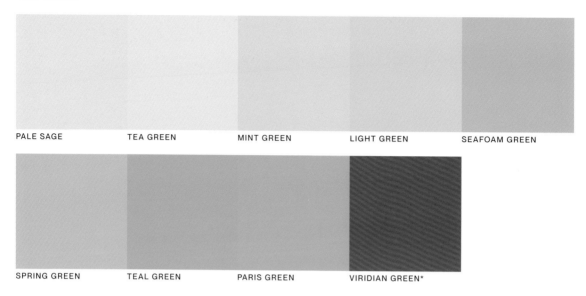

| PALE SAGE | TEA GREEN | MINT GREEN | LIGHT GREEN | SEAFOAM GREEN |

| SPRING GREEN | TEAL GREEN | PARIS GREEN | VIRIDIAN GREEN* |

Cyan and blue

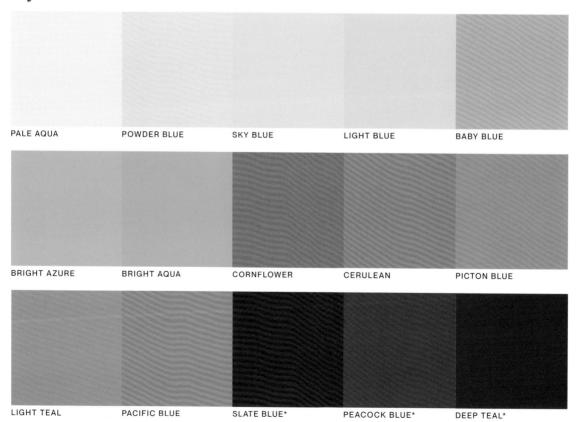

| PALE AQUA | POWDER BLUE | SKY BLUE | LIGHT BLUE | BABY BLUE |

| BRIGHT AZURE | BRIGHT AQUA | CORNFLOWER | CERULEAN | PICTON BLUE |

| LIGHT TEAL | PACIFIC BLUE | SLATE BLUE* | PEACOCK BLUE* | DEEP TEAL* |

Violet

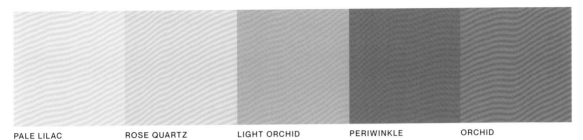

PALE LILAC   ROSE QUARTZ   LIGHT ORCHID   PERIWINKLE   ORCHID

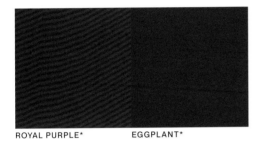

ROYAL PURPLE*   EGGPLANT*

Neutrals

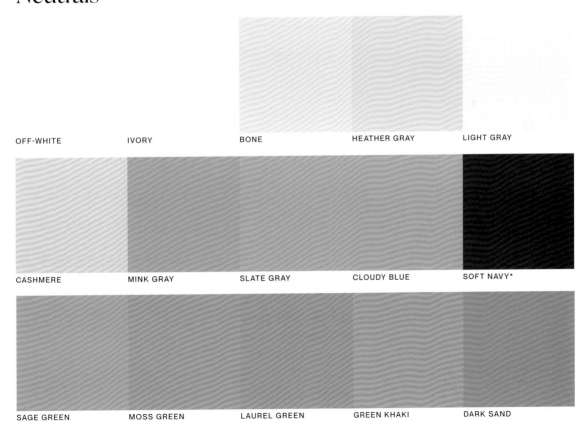

OFF-WHITE   IVORY   BONE   HEATHER GRAY   LIGHT GRAY

CASHMERE   MINK GRAY   SLATE GRAY   CLOUDY BLUE   SOFT NAVY*

SAGE GREEN   MOSS GREEN   LAUREL GREEN   GREEN KHAKI   DARK SAND

TRUE SUMMER

Color essence Cool and serene
Best colors Cool Dimmed Tones and Moderates

As a True Summer, your coloring is the classic representation of the muted, icy Summer palette. Your color essence is 100 percent cool and serene. It is a myth that the archetypal True Summer has blue eyes and ash-blond hair—brown eyes and deeper hair levels are far more common, and many True Summers have medium or deeper skin tones. What truly characterizes members of this season is their undertone, which contains very little to no signs of warmth, paired with a distinctly muted complexion.

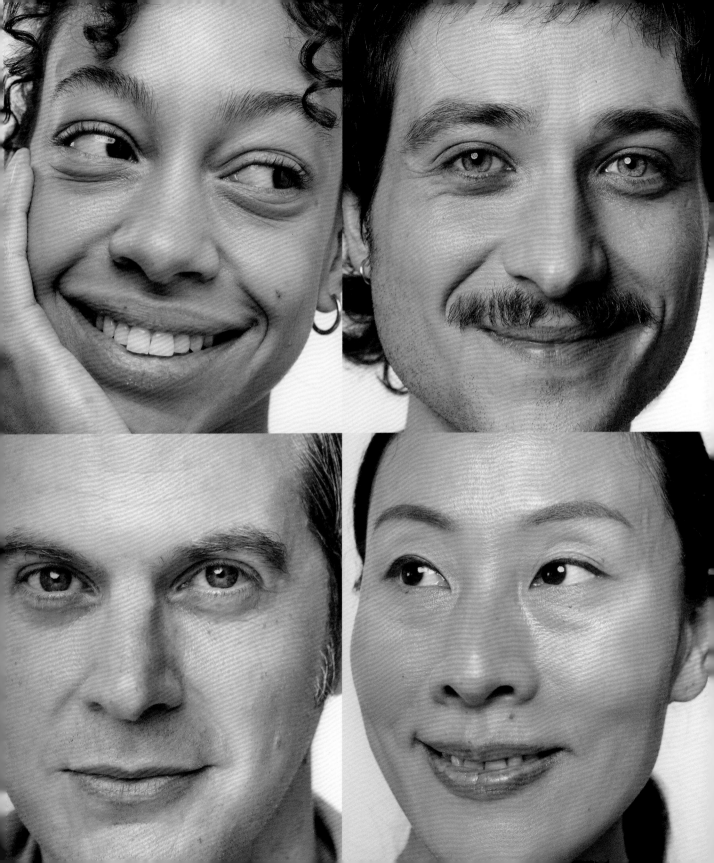

Your best colors

Like all true seasons, your undertone is clearly pronounced, which gives you a little less flexibility when it comes to the hue of your colors. Your palette only consists of cool and cool-neutral shades since even subtly warm shades will visibly clash with your complexion.

With a medium value and soft chroma, Dimmed Tones are a perfect match for your coloring. Moderates work just as well. If your skin tone is light-medium or deeper, you can also rock Dusky Shades. Here are some examples of shades that look great on True Summers:

Cool Dimmed Tones

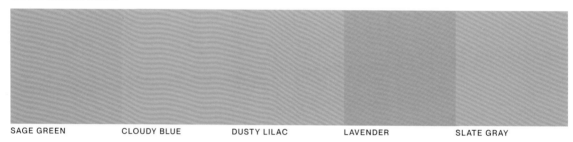

SAGE GREEN   CLOUDY BLUE   DUSTY LILAC   LAVENDER   SLATE GRAY

Cool Moderates

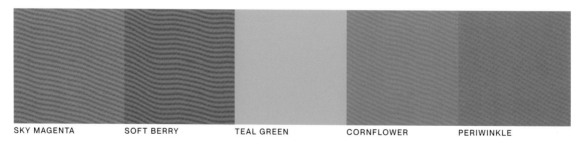

SKY MAGENTA   SOFT BERRY   TEAL GREEN   CORNFLOWER   PERIWINKLE

Cool Dusky Shades (*light-medium or deeper skin tones*)

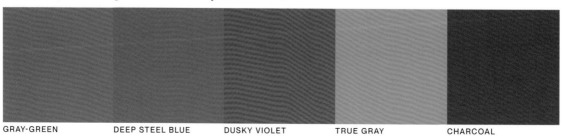

GRAY-GREEN   DEEP STEEL BLUE   DUSKY VIOLET   TRUE GRAY   CHARCOAL

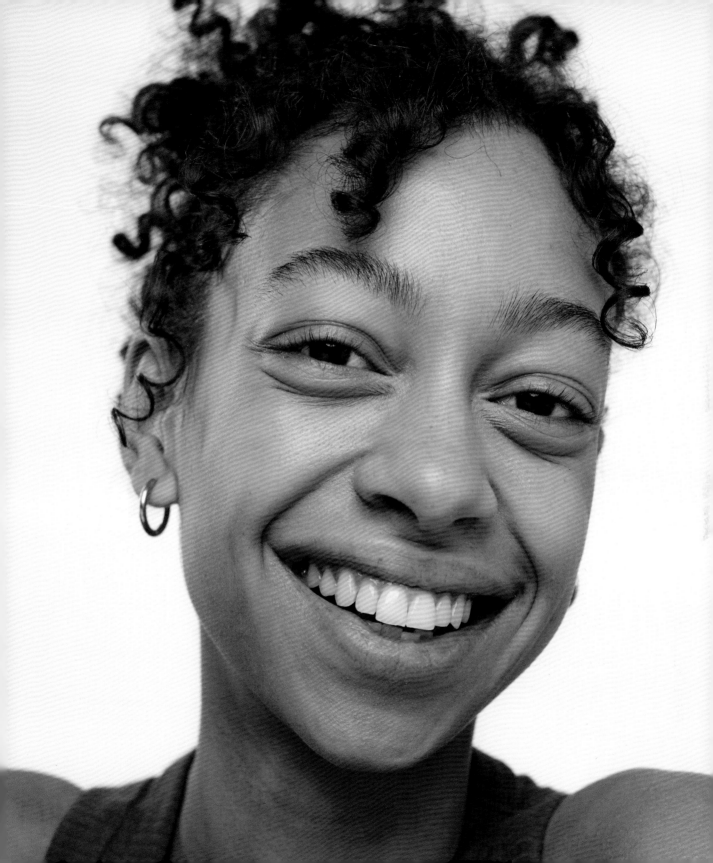

Levels of harmony

True Summers shine in cool-toned Moderates and Dimmed Tones. These two color genres make up the bulk of your color palette. But there are two other color genres you may want to try: Pastels and Pale Tones. Both are a tad too light to be a perfect match for True Summers, but in their cool versions, they will still look harmonious and can add some variety to your look. As one of the coolest seasons, True Summers have a low tolerance for any amount of warmth. Even warm-neutral shades are likely going to look dissonant. Here is an overview of how different undertones and color genres work on True Summers. Ratings for color genres are based on shades that match your best undertone (cool). Shades in other undertones will be less harmonious.

	Color genre	Undertone
PERFECT MATCH	Moderates Dimmed Tones Dusky Shades *(light-medium or deeper skin tones)*	Cool
HARMONIOUS	Pale Tones Pastels Rich Shades *(light-medium or deeper skin tones)*	Cool-neutral
OKAY	Dusky Shades *(fair or light skin tones)* Rich Shades *(fair or light skin tones)*	
DISSONANT	Jewel Tones	Warm-neutral
CLASH	Vivids Brights	Warm

Your "opposite" colors

Warm Brights and Vivids are your least harmonious colors. They don't echo any aspect of your coloring, and may clash with your complexion. Here are some examples:

Warm Brights

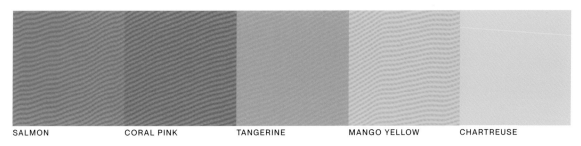

| SALMON | CORAL PINK | TANGERINE | MANGO YELLOW | CHARTREUSE |

Warm Vivids

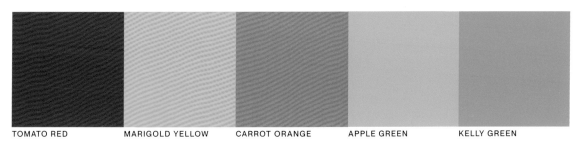

| TOMATO RED | MARIGOLD YELLOW | CARROT ORANGE | APPLE GREEN | KELLY GREEN |

How aging may affect your best colors

Like all seasons, True Summers lose some of their chroma and contrast with age. This means that the Moderates in your palette may start to look slightly less harmonious, while Pale Tones may become more harmonious. The undertone of your best colors will remain stable throughout your life.

How a suntan may affect your best colors

If your skin tone is fair or light, a strong suntan will warm up your complexion. As a result, warm-neutral hues will likely appear okay instead of dissonant. Regardless of your skin tone, a strong suntan will also increase your chroma somewhat, making Pastels a perfect match for you.

Best colors by hue

Since True Summers don't do well with warmth, not all hue families are featured in your palette. This includes yellow and orange hues, which are inherently warm, and brown and beige shades, which are desaturated versions of orange hues. But your palette does include a range of shades that wash out pretty much everyone else, including true grayscale shades, silver, blue-toned pinks, and periwinkles.

This section will look at your full color palette, broken down by hue. We will cover hair colors, makeup, and jewelry in later chapters! The True Summer palette includes a range of Dusky Shades and Rich Shades, marked with an asterisk. These are a perfect match or harmonious on skin tones that are light-medium or deeper.

Red and pink

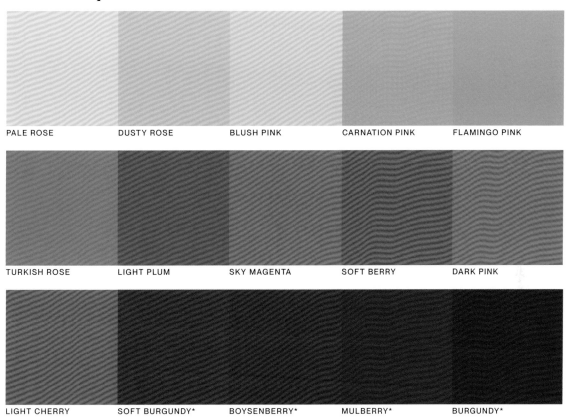

PALE ROSE	DUSTY ROSE	BLUSH PINK	CARNATION PINK	FLAMINGO PINK
TURKISH ROSE	LIGHT PLUM	SKY MAGENTA	SOFT BERRY	DARK PINK
LIGHT CHERRY	SOFT BURGUNDY*	BOYSENBERRY*	MULBERRY*	BURGUNDY*

Green

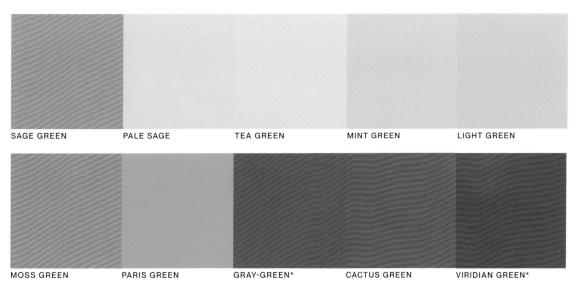

SAGE GREEN	PALE SAGE	TEA GREEN	MINT GREEN	LIGHT GREEN
MOSS GREEN	PARIS GREEN	GRAY-GREEN*	CACTUS GREEN	VIRIDIAN GREEN*

Cyan and blue

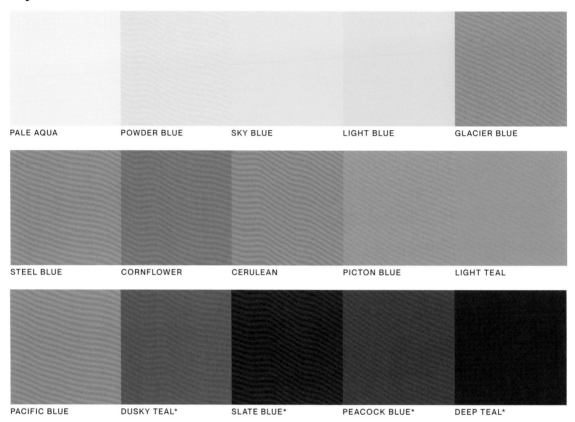

PALE AQUA	POWDER BLUE	SKY BLUE	LIGHT BLUE	GLACIER BLUE
STEEL BLUE	CORNFLOWER	CERULEAN	PICTON BLUE	LIGHT TEAL
PACIFIC BLUE	DUSKY TEAL*	SLATE BLUE*	PEACOCK BLUE*	DEEP TEAL*

Violet

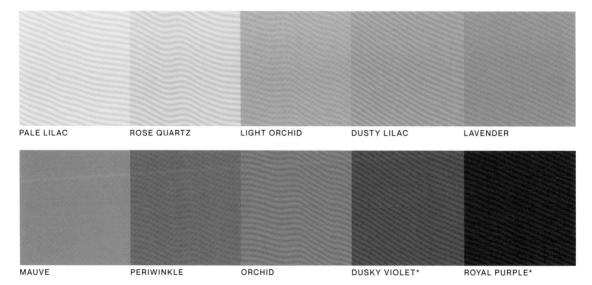

PALE LILAC	ROSE QUARTZ	LIGHT ORCHID	DUSTY LILAC	LAVENDER
MAUVE	PERIWINKLE	ORCHID	DUSKY VIOLET*	ROYAL PURPLE*

Neutrals

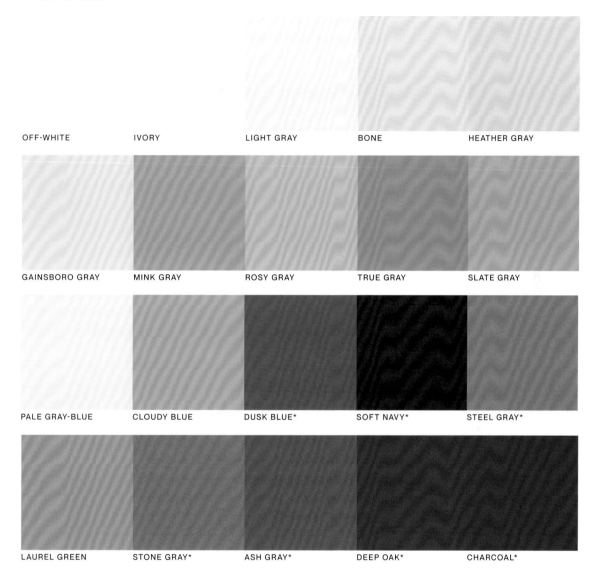

OFF-WHITE	IVORY	LIGHT GRAY	BONE	HEATHER GRAY
GAINSBORO GRAY	MINK GRAY	ROSY GRAY	TRUE GRAY	SLATE GRAY
PALE GRAY-BLUE	CLOUDY BLUE	DUSK BLUE*	SOFT NAVY*	STEEL GRAY*
LAUREL GREEN	STONE GRAY*	ASH GRAY*	DEEP OAK*	CHARCOAL*

SOFT SUMMER

Color essence Serene and subdued
Best colors Cool-neutral Dimmed Tones and Dusky Shades

Like all Summers, your coloring is characteristically muted and cool. But as a Soft Summer, you also have a touch of Autumn. The result is a much deeper, earthier version of the classic Summer palette. Think less pastel-candy hues, and more olive shades, dusky blues, and stoney grays.

Compared to other Summer seasons, Soft Summers have considerable contrast and usually have deeper features. Even lighter-skinned Soft Summers can pull off quite a bit of depth.

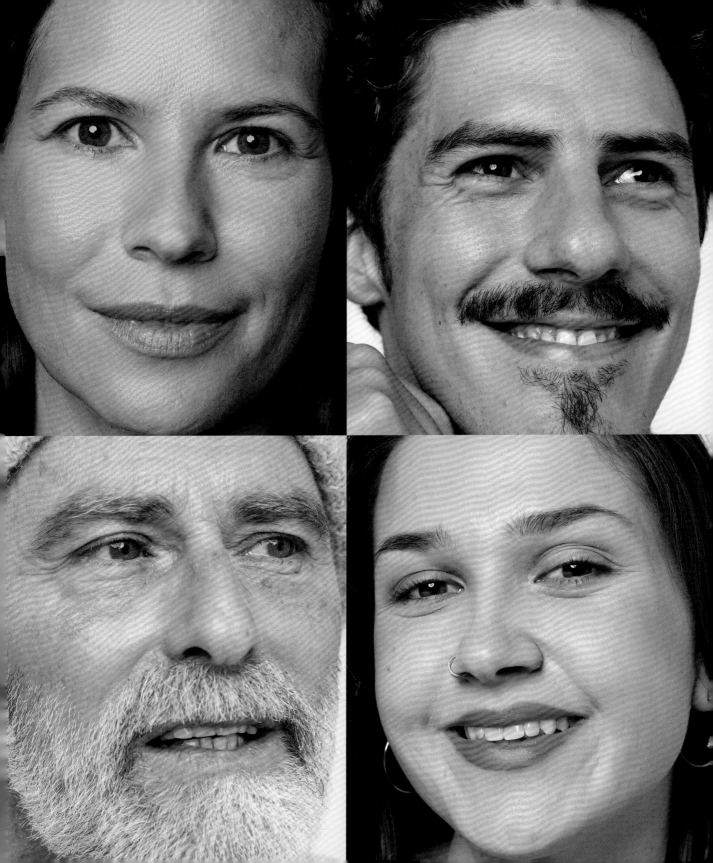

Your best colors

All Soft Summers do better with deeper rather than lighter shades—a key characteristic that separates you from other Summer types. As a soft season, you cannot handle a lot of saturation; your best colors all have a soft chroma. Your best color genres are Dimmed Tones and Dusky Shades.

Across all color genres, you look best in cool-neutral shades. Cool shades will work better than warm-neutral colors.

Here are some examples of your best color genres in cool-neutral versions:

Cool-neutral Dimmed Tones

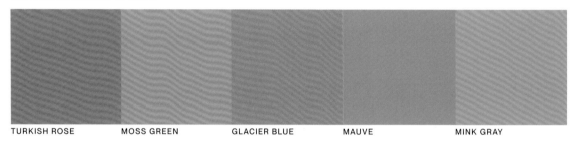

TURKISH ROSE   MOSS GREEN   GLACIER BLUE   MAUVE   MINK GRAY

Cool-neutral Dusky Shades

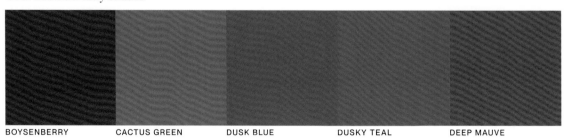

BOYSENBERRY   CACTUS GREEN   DUSK BLUE   DUSKY TEAL   DEEP MAUVE

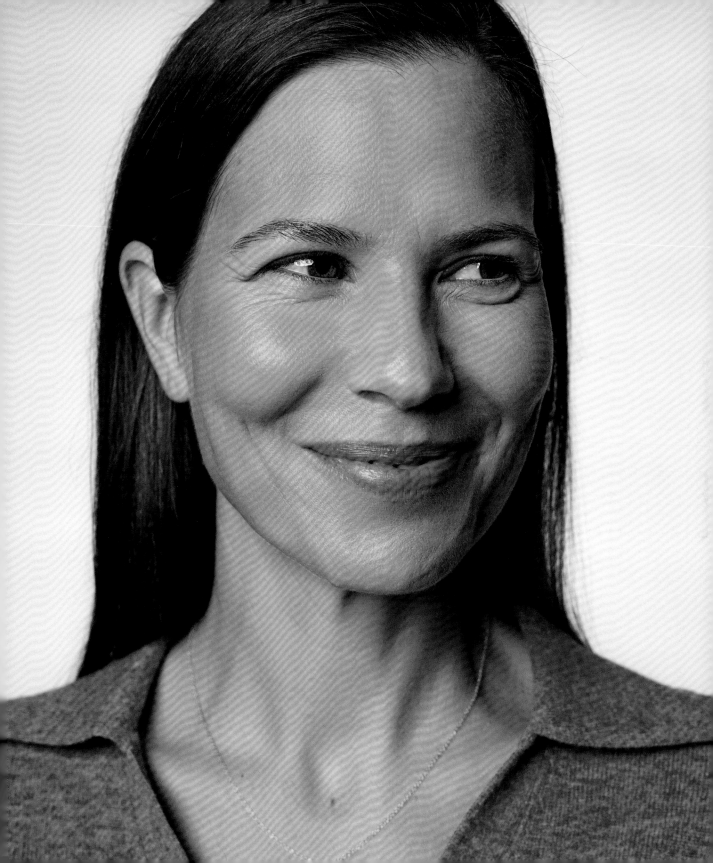

Levels of harmony

As a Soft Summer, your best colors are cool-neutral Dimmed Tones and Dusky Shades, but remember: color harmony comes in levels! Two other color genres, Moderates and Rich Shades, may not fit your color dimensions perfectly, but they still complement your coloring reasonably well in their cool-neutral versions.

Here is an overview of how different undertones and color genres work on Soft Summers. Ratings for color genres are based on shades that match your best undertone (cool-neutral). Shades in other undertones will be less harmonious.

	Color genre	Undertone
PERFECT MATCH	Dimmed Tones Dusky Shades	Cool-neutral
HARMONIOUS	Rich Shades Moderates	Cool
OKAY	Pale Tones	Warm-neutral
DISSONANT	Jewel Tones Pastels	Warm
CLASH	Brights Vivids	

Your "opposite" colors

Warm Brights and Vivids are your least harmonious colors. They don't echo any aspect of your coloring, and may clash with your complexion. Here are some examples:

Warm Brights

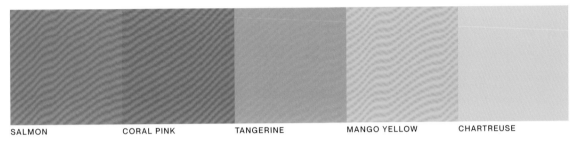

| SALMON | CORAL PINK | TANGERINE | MANGO YELLOW | CHARTREUSE |

Warm Vivids

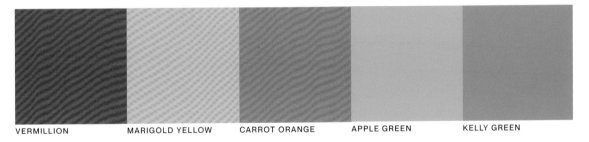

| VERMILLION | MARIGOLD YELLOW | CARROT ORANGE | APPLE GREEN | KELLY GREEN |

How aging may affect your best colors

Like all seasons, Soft Summers lose some of their chroma and contrast with age. This means that the Rich Shades and Moderates in your palette may start to look slightly less harmonious, while Dimmed Tones may become even more harmonious. The undertone of your best colors will remain stable throughout your life.

How a suntan may affect your best colors

If your skin tone is fair or light, a strong suntan will warm up your complexion. As a result, warm-neutral hues will likely appear harmonious instead of okay. Regardless of your skin tone, a strong suntan will also increase your chroma somewhat, making Moderates a perfect match for you.

Best colors by hue

The Soft Summer palette is dusky, gentle, and deep. Although your undertone is cool-neutral, your palette appears quite cool because of its low chroma (grayscale shades are 100 percent cool). Despite your cool-neutral undertone, any warmth will likely clash with your complexion. Because of this, your palette does not include yellow, orange, or brown, as these are inherently warm.

This section will look at your full color palette, broken down by hue. Note that we will cover hair colors, makeup, and jewelry in later chapters!

Red and pink

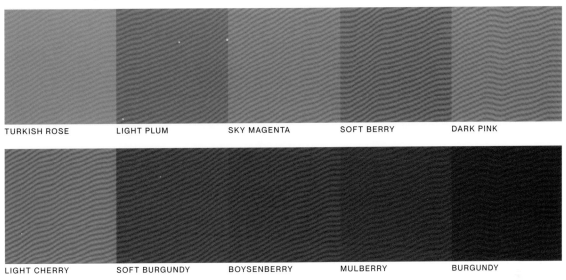

TURKISH ROSE LIGHT PLUM SKY MAGENTA SOFT BERRY DARK PINK

LIGHT CHERRY SOFT BURGUNDY BOYSENBERRY MULBERRY BURGUNDY

Green

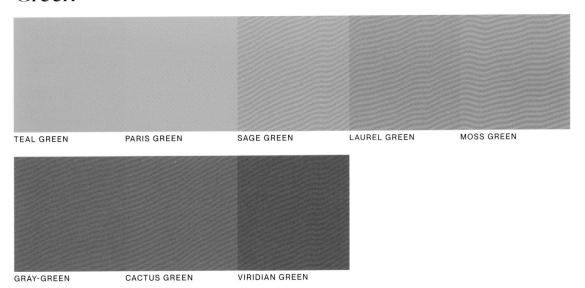

TEAL GREEN PARIS GREEN SAGE GREEN LAUREL GREEN MOSS GREEN

GRAY-GREEN CACTUS GREEN VIRIDIAN GREEN

Cyan and blue

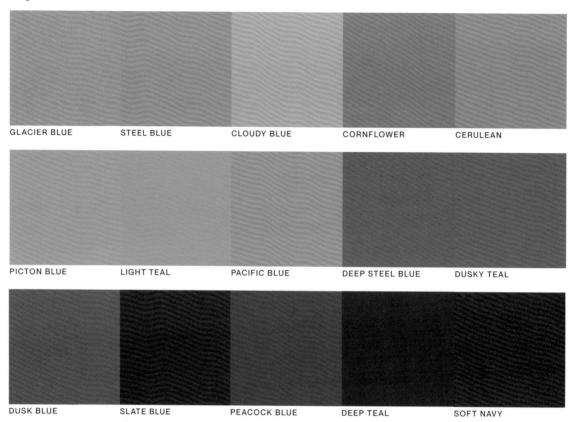

GLACIER BLUE	STEEL BLUE	CLOUDY BLUE	CORNFLOWER	CERULEAN
PICTON BLUE	LIGHT TEAL	PACIFIC BLUE	DEEP STEEL BLUE	DUSKY TEAL
DUSK BLUE	SLATE BLUE	PEACOCK BLUE	DEEP TEAL	SOFT NAVY

Violet

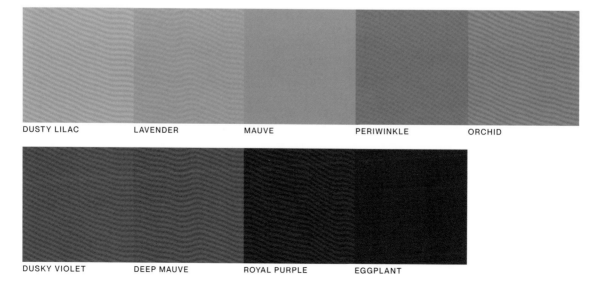

DUSTY LILAC	LAVENDER	MAUVE	PERIWINKLE	ORCHID
DUSKY VIOLET	DEEP MAUVE	ROYAL PURPLE	EGGPLANT	

Neutrals

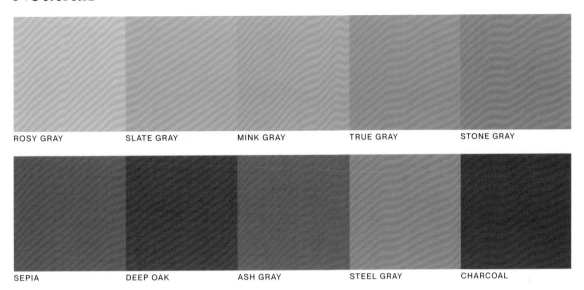

ROSY GRAY   SLATE GRAY   MINK GRAY   TRUE GRAY   STONE GRAY

SEPIA   DEEP OAK   ASH GRAY   STEEL GRAY   CHARCOAL

SOFT AUTUMN

Color essence Soft and earthy
Best colors Warm-neutral Dimmed Tones and Dusky Shades

You hail from the Autumn family tree and your coloring is characteristically warm and muted. But unlike the other Autumn types, you also have a bit of Summer. That Summer influence acts like a hazy filter over your rich, velvety Autumn base, toning down your warmth and reducing your contrast. The result is a super soft, earthy color essence that is reminiscent of the first days of autumn.

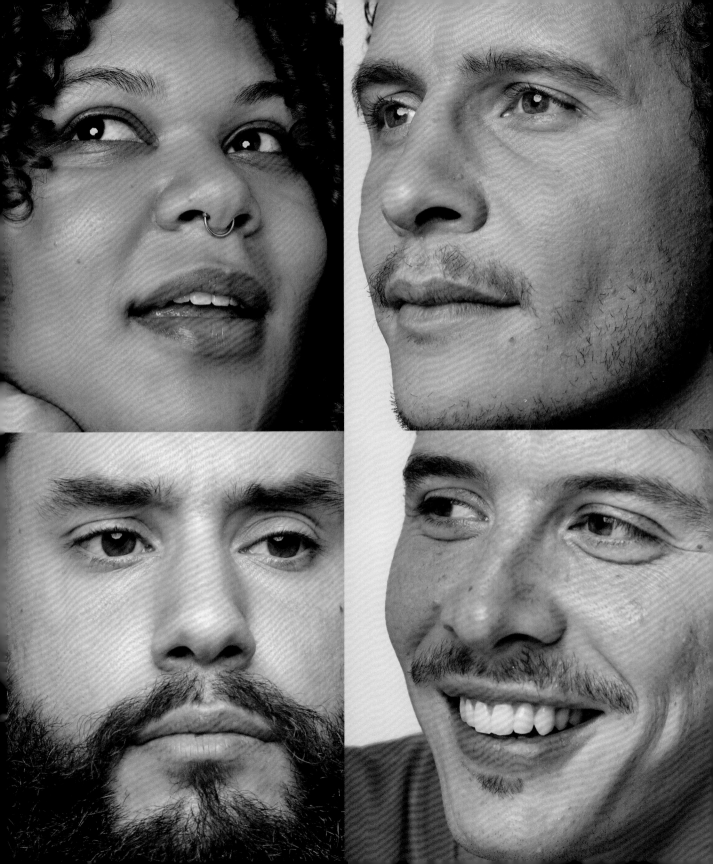

Your best colors

As a Soft Autumn, you are probably drawn to calmer, slightly deeper shades. Your best color genres are Dimmed Tones and Dusky Shades. Regardless of skin tone, Soft Autumns don't do well with light colors and anything too vibrant.

Across all color genres, warm-neutral shades are the best fit for your undertone. Here are some shades you'll look fabulous in:

Warm-neutral Dimmed Tones

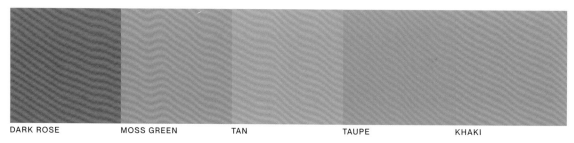

| DARK ROSE | MOSS GREEN | TAN | TAUPE | KHAKI |

Warm-neutral Dusky Shades

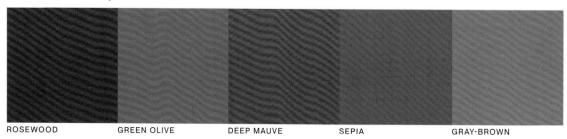

| ROSEWOOD | GREEN OLIVE | DEEP MAUVE | SEPIA | GRAY-BROWN |

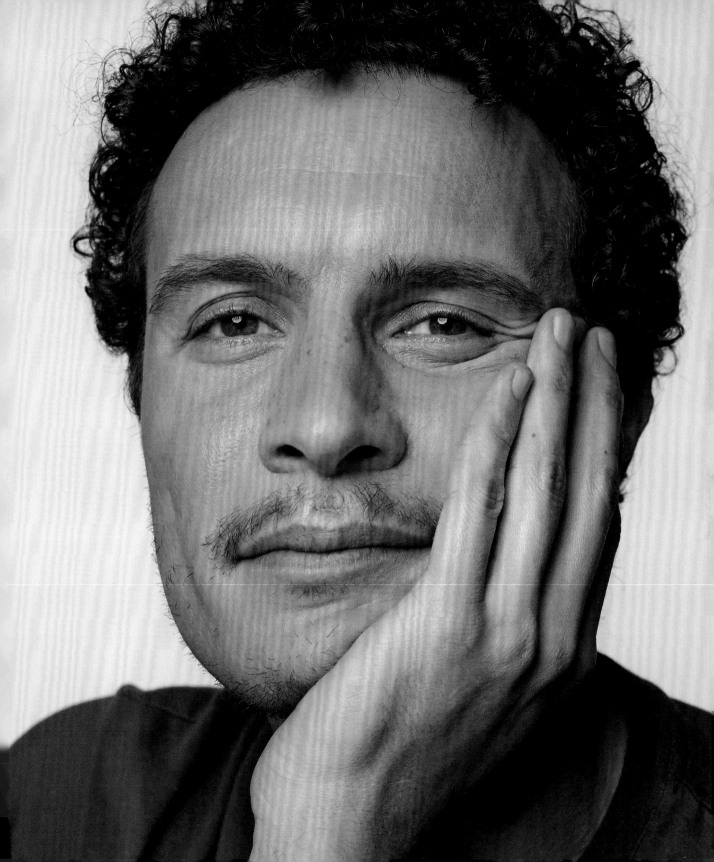

Levels of harmony

Although your best colors are warm-neutral Dimmed Tones and Dusky Shades, other types of colors will also look harmonious. As a warm-neutral season, you are quite flexible when it comes to the undertone of your colors. While warm-neutral shades work best, your palette also includes several warm and even cool-neutral colors, since these will still look harmonious on you.

When it comes to color genres, also consider Moderates and Rich Shades. These can be a little intense on your coloring, but in warm-neutral versions, they will still look good.

	Color genre	Undertone
PERFECT MATCH	Dimmed Tones Dusky Shades	Warm-neutral
HARMONIOUS	Rich Shades Moderates	Warm Cool-neutral
OKAY	Pale Tones	Cool
DISSONANT	Jewel Tones Pastels	
CLASH	Vivids Brights	

On the opposite page is an overview of how well different undertones and color genres work on Soft Autumns. Ratings for color genres are based on shades that match your best undertone (warm-neutral). Shades in other undertones will be less harmonious.

Your "opposite" colors

Cool Brights and Vivids are your least harmonious colors. They don't echo any aspect of your coloring, and may clash with your complexion. Here are some examples:

Cool Brights

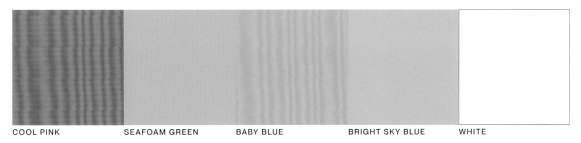

| COOL PINK | SEAFOAM GREEN | BABY BLUE | BRIGHT SKY BLUE | WHITE |

Cool Vivids

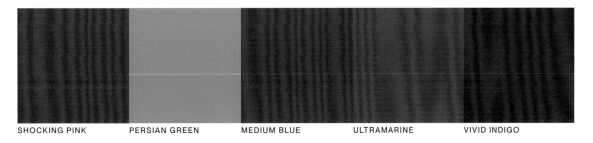

| SHOCKING PINK | PERSIAN GREEN | MEDIUM BLUE | ULTRAMARINE | VIVID INDIGO |

How aging may affect your best colors

Like all seasons, Soft Autumns lose some of their chroma and contrast with age. This means that the Rich Shades in your palette may start to look slightly less harmonious, while Dimmed Tones may become even more harmonious. The undertone of your best colors will remain stable throughout your life.

How a suntan may affect your best colors

If your skin tone is fair or light, a strong suntan will warm up your complexion. As a result, you'll likely do just as well with warm hues as with warm-neutral ones. Regardless of your skin tone, a strong suntan will also increase your chroma somewhat, allowing you to pull off Moderates, making them a perfect match for you.

Best colors by hue

This section will look at your full color palette, broken down by hue. Note that we will cover hair colors, makeup, and jewelry in later chapters!

Red and pink

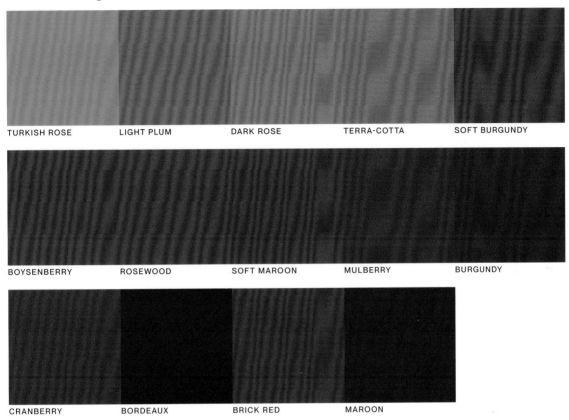

| TURKISH ROSE | LIGHT PLUM | DARK ROSE | TERRA-COTTA | SOFT BURGUNDY |

| BOYSENBERRY | ROSEWOOD | SOFT MAROON | MULBERRY | BURGUNDY |

| CRANBERRY | BORDEAUX | BRICK RED | MAROON |

Orange and yellow

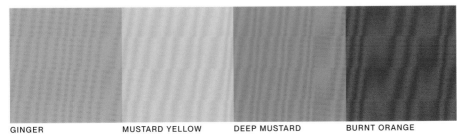

| GINGER | MUSTARD YELLOW | DEEP MUSTARD | BURNT ORANGE |

Green

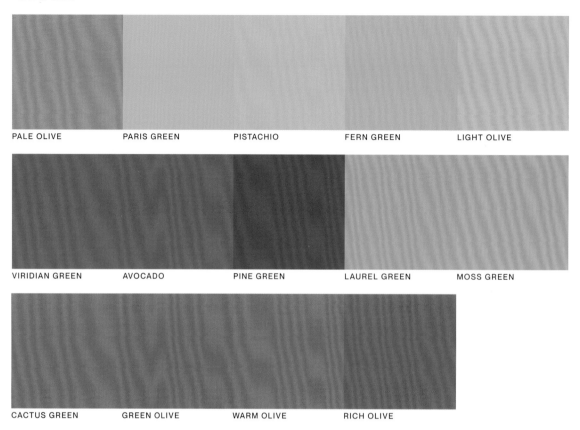

PALE OLIVE	PARIS GREEN	PISTACHIO	FERN GREEN	LIGHT OLIVE
VIRIDIAN GREEN	AVOCADO	PINE GREEN	LAUREL GREEN	MOSS GREEN
CACTUS GREEN	GREEN OLIVE	WARM OLIVE	RICH OLIVE	

Cyan and blue

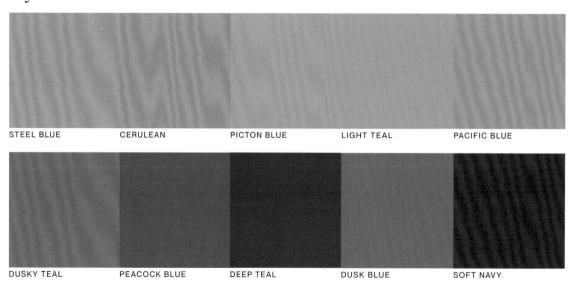

| STEEL BLUE | CERULEAN | PICTON BLUE | LIGHT TEAL | PACIFIC BLUE |
| DUSKY TEAL | PEACOCK BLUE | DEEP TEAL | DUSK BLUE | SOFT NAVY |

Violet

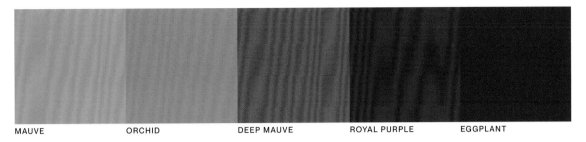

MAUVE ORCHID DEEP MAUVE ROYAL PURPLE EGGPLANT

Neutrals

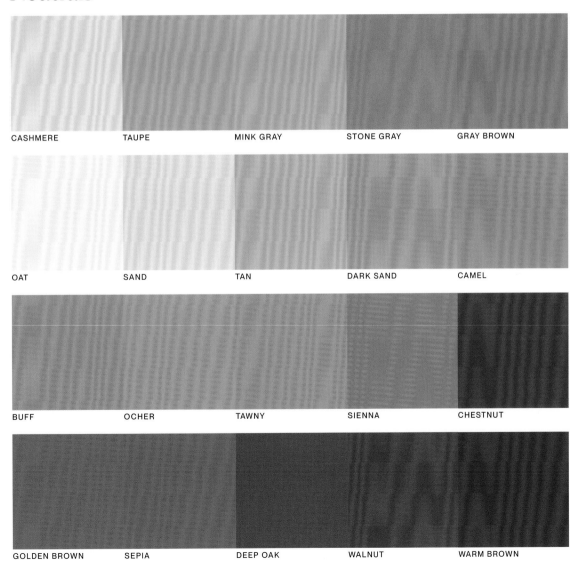

CASHMERE TAUPE MINK GRAY STONE GRAY GRAY BROWN

OAT SAND TAN DARK SAND CAMEL

BUFF OCHER TAWNY SIENNA CHESTNUT

GOLDEN BROWN SEPIA DEEP OAK WALNUT WARM BROWN

TRUE AUTUMN

Color essence Warm and rich
Best colors Warm Dusky Shades
and Rich Shades

PERSONAL COLOR

As a True Autumn, your color essence is rich, earthy, and velvety.
You are the warmest and also the rarest of the Autumn seasons.
The True Autumn complexion is warm, golden, soft, and blended
regardless of skin tone. You have a lot of contrast and do better with
deeper, richer shades than pale Pastels. You probably don't love
pinks on your complexion and haven't met a shade of brown that
doesn't work on you.

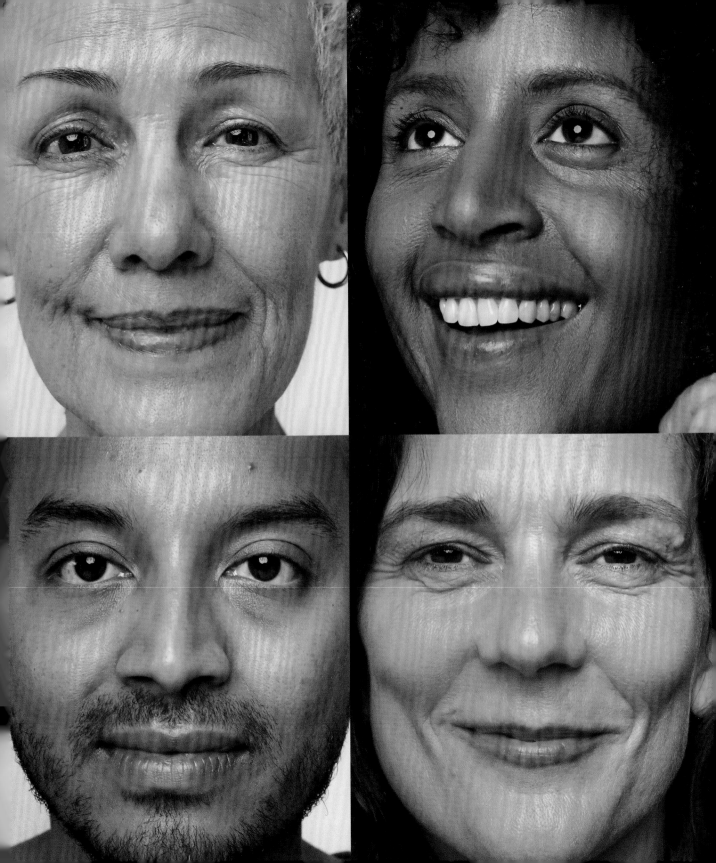

Your best colors

As a high-contrast, soft season, True Autumns look amazing in Dusky and Rich Shades: deeper color genres that aren't too vibrant.

Across all color genres, warm shades best harmonize with your warm undertone. These are some shades that True Autumns like you shine in:

Warm Dimmed Tones

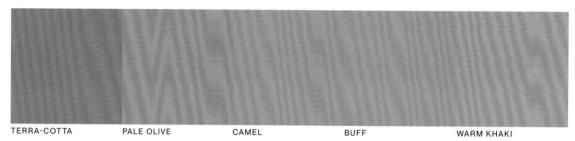

TERRA-COTTA   PALE OLIVE   CAMEL   BUFF   WARM KHAKI

Warm Dusky Shades

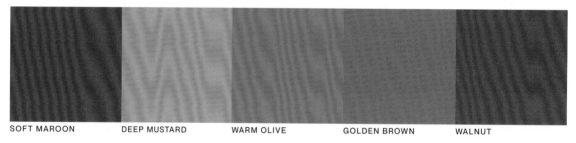

SOFT MAROON   DEEP MUSTARD   WARM OLIVE   GOLDEN BROWN   WALNUT

Warm Rich Shades

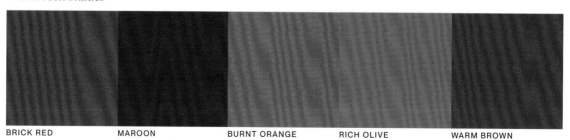

BRICK RED   MAROON   BURNT ORANGE   RICH OLIVE   WARM BROWN

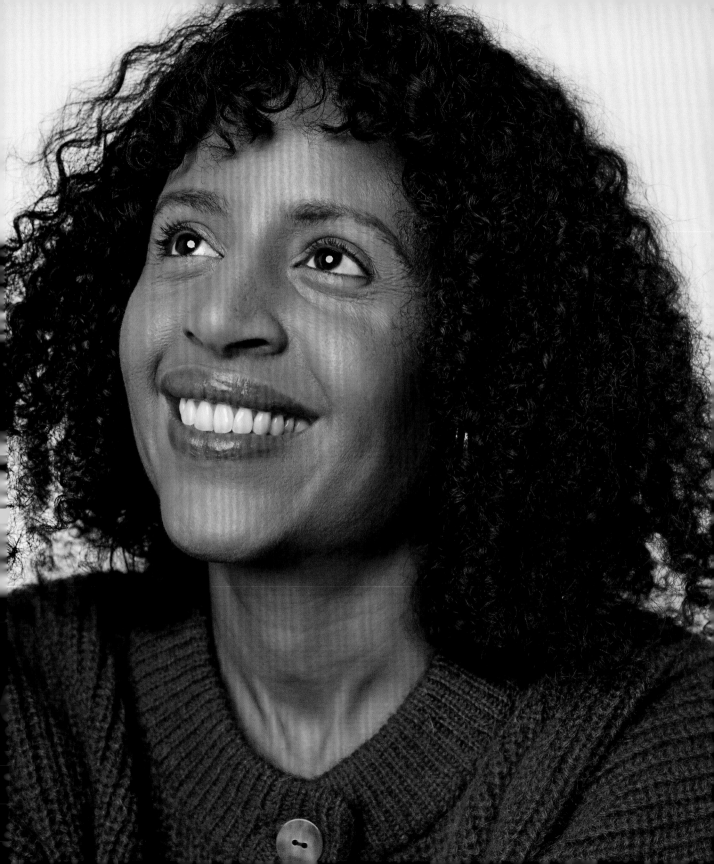

Levels of harmony

Warm Dusky and Rich Shades best complement the True Autumn complexion. But what about other colors? Color harmony comes in levels: Just because a particular shade is not a perfect fit for your coloring does not mean it will look dissonant. Dimmed Tones are a touch lighter than your best color genres but equally muted so tend to work well, too. Jewel Tones may look a little intense on you, but as long as they match your undertone (warm), they will still look harmonious.

When it comes to the undertone of your colors, there is no such thing as a "too warm" shade. Warm-neutral shades will also look great on you, and your palette even includes a few cool-neutral colors! These won't be anything to write home about, but they won't look bad (warm seasons tend to have a much higher tolerance for cool shades than

	Color genre	Undertone
PERFECT MATCH	Dusky Shades Rich Shades	Warm
HARMONIOUS	Dimmed Tones Jewel Tones	Warm-neutral
OKAY	Moderates	Cool-neutral
DISSONANT	Vivids Pastels	Cool
CLASH	Pale Tones Brights	

vice versa). Only cool shades won't mesh well with your coloring, so your palette does not include grayscale shades or pure black.

On the left is an overview of how well different undertones and color genres work on True Autumns. Ratings for color genres are based on shades that match your best undertone (warm). Shades in other undertones will be less harmonious.

Your "opposite" colors

Cool Pale Tones and Brights are your least harmonious colors. They don't echo any aspect of your coloring, and may clash with your complexion. Here are some examples:

Cool Pale Tones

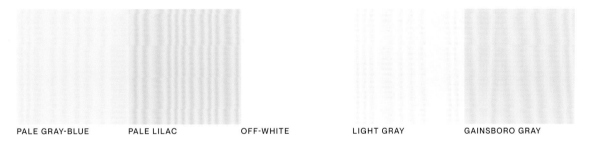

PALE GRAY-BLUE   PALE LILAC   OFF-WHITE   LIGHT GRAY   GAINSBORO GRAY

Cool Brights

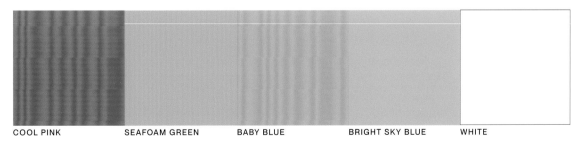

COOL PINK   SEAFOAM GREEN   BABY BLUE   BRIGHT SKY BLUE   WHITE

How aging may affect your best colors

Like all seasons, True Autumns lose some of their chroma and contrast with age. This means that the Jewel Tones in your palette may start to look slightly less harmonious, while Dimmed Tones may become more harmonious. As a warm season, your undertone may also become slightly less pronounced with age, and you may gravitate to warm-neutral colors.

How a suntan may affect your best colors

If your skin tone is fair or light, a strong suntan will warm up your complexion, allowing you to truly rock the warmest shades of your palette. Regardless of your skin tone, a strong suntan will also increase your chroma somewhat, allowing you to pull off Moderates.

Best colors by hue

This section will look at your full color palette, broken down by hue. Note that we will cover hair colors, makeup, and jewelry in later chapters!

Red and pink

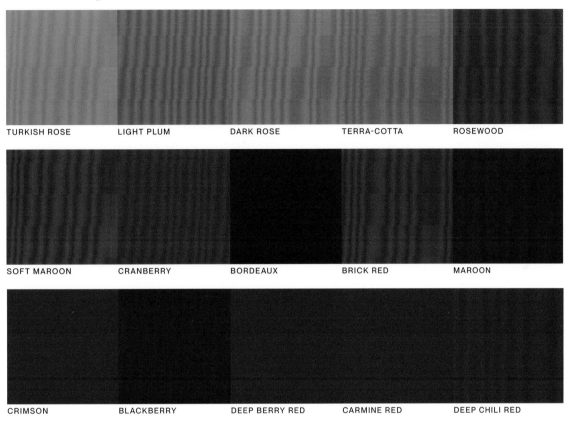

TURKISH ROSE	LIGHT PLUM	DARK ROSE	TERRA-COTTA	ROSEWOOD
SOFT MAROON	CRANBERRY	BORDEAUX	BRICK RED	MAROON
CRIMSON	BLACKBERRY	DEEP BERRY RED	CARMINE RED	DEEP CHILI RED

Orange and yellow

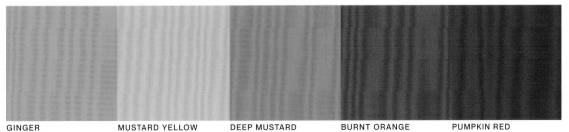

GINGER	MUSTARD YELLOW	DEEP MUSTARD	BURNT ORANGE	PUMPKIN RED

Green

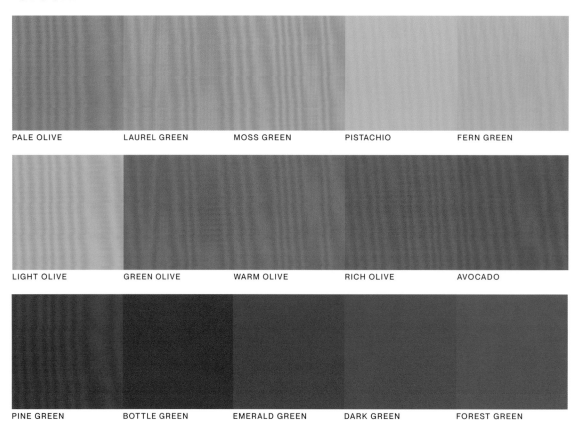

| PALE OLIVE | LAUREL GREEN | MOSS GREEN | PISTACHIO | FERN GREEN |

| LIGHT OLIVE | GREEN OLIVE | WARM OLIVE | RICH OLIVE | AVOCADO |

| PINE GREEN | BOTTLE GREEN | EMERALD GREEN | DARK GREEN | FOREST GREEN |

Cyan and blue

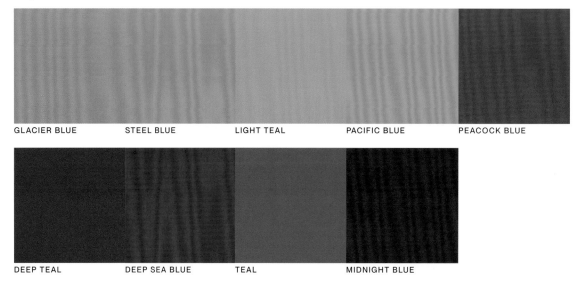

| GLACIER BLUE | STEEL BLUE | LIGHT TEAL | PACIFIC BLUE | PEACOCK BLUE |

| DEEP TEAL | DEEP SEA BLUE | TEAL | MIDNIGHT BLUE |

Violet

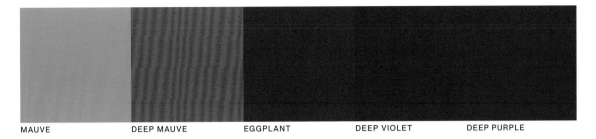

MAUVE   DEEP MAUVE   EGGPLANT   DEEP VIOLET   DEEP PURPLE

Neutrals

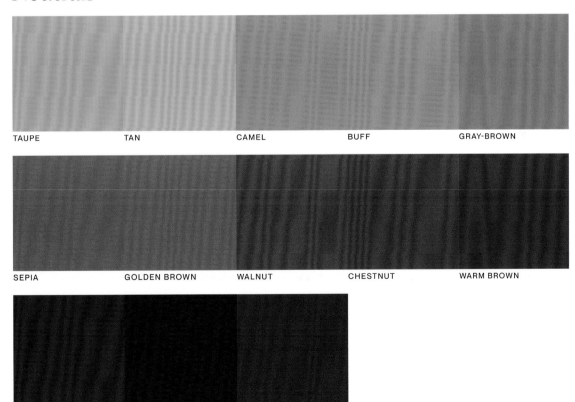

TAUPE   TAN   CAMEL   BUFF   GRAY-BROWN

SEPIA   GOLDEN BROWN   WALNUT   CHESTNUT   WARM BROWN

ESPRESSO   MAHOGANY   RUSSET

DEEP AUTUMN

Color essence Rich and intense

Best colors Warm-neutral Dusky Shades, Rich Shades, and Jewel Tones

As a Deep Autumn, your coloring is uniquely rich, intense, and characterized by contrast. Your color essence combines the Autumn season's earthy richness with the Winter season's brilliant intensity. The Deep Autumn palette is like the nighttime version of the classic, earthy Autumn palette: the shades are deeper, clearer, and not quite as warm.

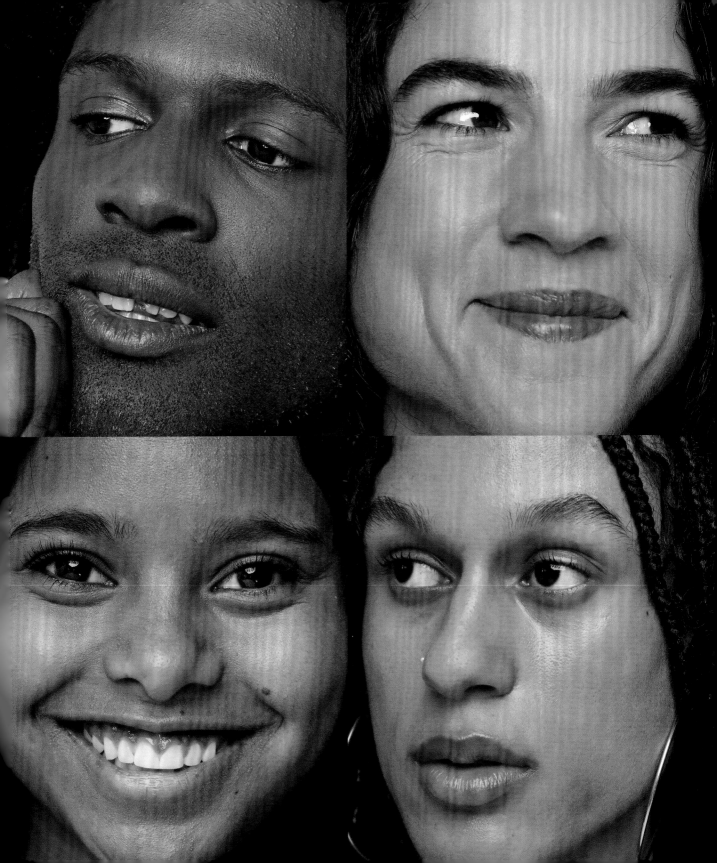

Your best colors

Like all Autumns, you suit warmer, deeper shades, but as a medium-chroma season, you can wear a much more comprehensive range of color genres than your softer Autumn sisters. Your best colors are, above all, deep. Dusky Shades, Rich Shades, and Jewel Tones: all three deep-value color genres echo your high-contrast coloring perfectly.

In terms of undertone, warm-neutral shades work best across all color genres. Here are some examples of colors that will look amazing on you:

Warm-neutral Dusky Shades

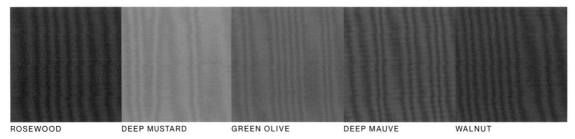

ROSEWOOD DEEP MUSTARD GREEN OLIVE DEEP MAUVE WALNUT

Warm-neutral Rich Shades

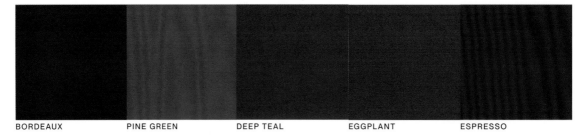

BORDEAUX PINE GREEN DEEP TEAL EGGPLANT ESPRESSO

Warm-neutral Jewel Tones

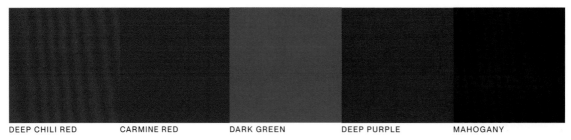

DEEP CHILI RED CARMINE RED DARK GREEN DEEP PURPLE MAHOGANY

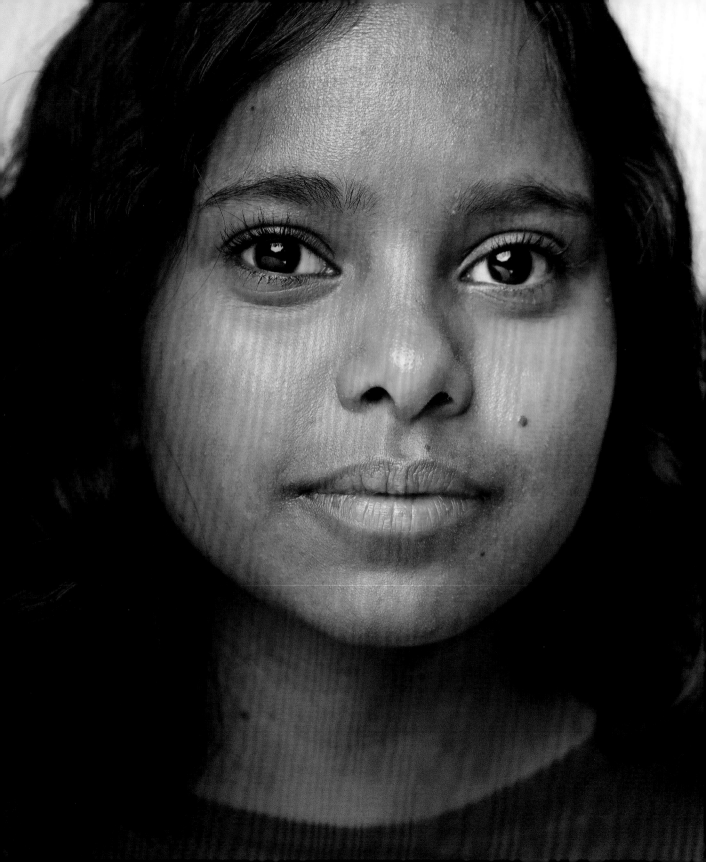

Levels of harmony

Your best colors are Dusky Shades, Rich Shades, and Jewel Tones with a warm-neutral undertone. But that does not mean all other colors will dull your shine. Due to your natural intensity, you can also pull off a staple from the Deep Winter's palette: Vivids.

Like all warm-neutral seasons, Deep Autumns are very versatile regarding the undertone of your colors. While warm-neutral shades work best, both warm and cool-neutral shades will still look harmonious. Only obviously cool shades may drag down your natural radiance a little.

Here is an overview of how well different undertones and color genres work on Deep Autumns. Ratings for color genres are based

	Color genre	Undertone
PERFECT MATCH	Dusky Shades Rich Shades Jewel Tones	Warm-neutral
HARMONIOUS	Vivids	Warm Cool-neutral
OKAY	Dimmed Tones	Cool
DISSONANT	Moderates Pastels	
CLASH	Brights Pale Tones	

on shades that match your best undertone (warm-neutral). Shades in other undertones will be less harmonious.

Your "opposite" colors

Cool Pale Tones and Brights are your least harmonious colors. They don't echo any aspect of your coloring, and may clash with your complexion. Here are some examples:

Cool Pale Tones

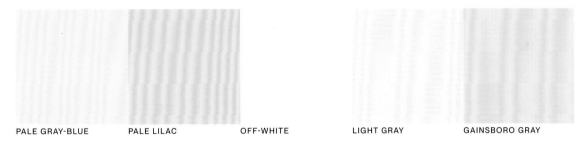

| PALE GRAY-BLUE | PALE LILAC | OFF-WHITE | LIGHT GRAY | GAINSBORO GRAY |

Cool Brights

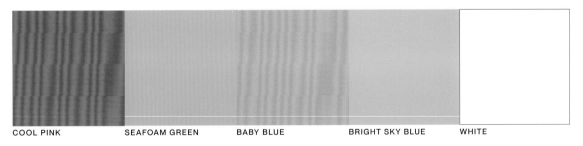

| COOL PINK | SEAFOAM GREEN | BABY BLUE | BRIGHT SKY BLUE | WHITE |

How aging may affect your best colors

Like all seasons, Deep Autumns lose some of their chroma and contrast with age. This means that the Vivids and Jewel Tones in your palette may start to look slightly less harmonious, while Dimmed Tones may become harmonious. The undertone of your best colors will remain stable throughout your life.

How a suntan may affect your best colors

If your skin tone is fair or light, a strong suntan will warm up your complexion. As a result, you'll likely do just as well with warm hues as with warm-neutral ones. Regardless of your skin tone, a strong suntan will also increase your chroma somewhat, making Vivids a perfect match for you.

Best colors by hue

This section will look at your full color palette, broken down by hue. Note that we will cover hair colors, makeup, and jewelry in later chapters!

Red and pink

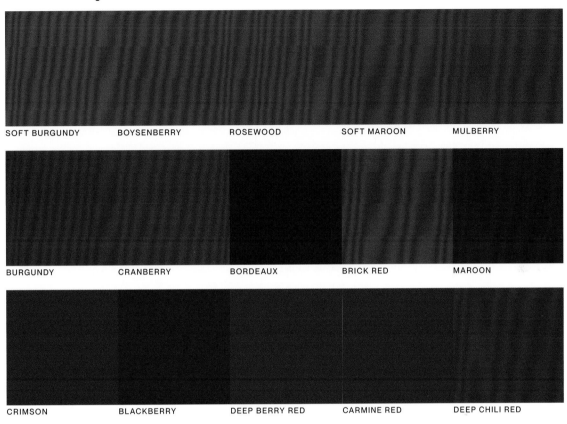

| SOFT BURGUNDY | BOYSENBERRY | ROSEWOOD | SOFT MAROON | MULBERRY |

| BURGUNDY | CRANBERRY | BORDEAUX | BRICK RED | MAROON |

| CRIMSON | BLACKBERRY | DEEP BERRY RED | CARMINE RED | DEEP CHILI RED |

Orange and yellow

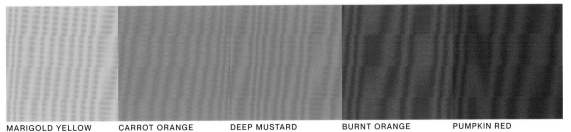

| MARIGOLD YELLOW | CARROT ORANGE | DEEP MUSTARD | BURNT ORANGE | PUMPKIN RED |

Green

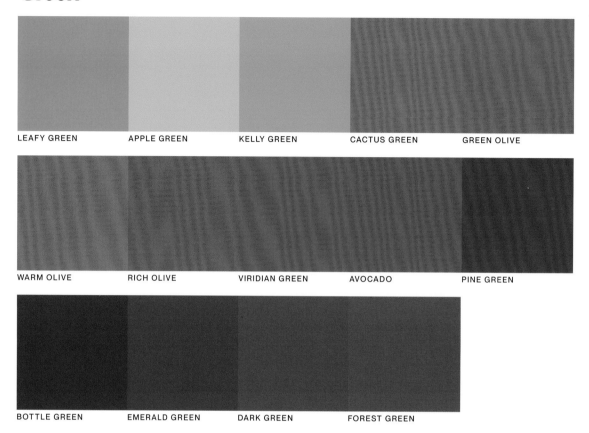

LEAFY GREEN   APPLE GREEN   KELLY GREEN   CACTUS GREEN   GREEN OLIVE

WARM OLIVE   RICH OLIVE   VIRIDIAN GREEN   AVOCADO   PINE GREEN

BOTTLE GREEN   EMERALD GREEN   DARK GREEN   FOREST GREEN

Cyan and blue

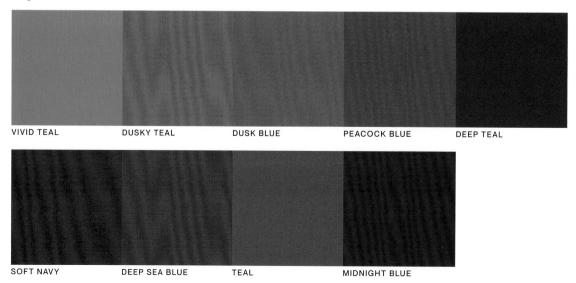

VIVID TEAL   DUSKY TEAL   DUSK BLUE   PEACOCK BLUE   DEEP TEAL

SOFT NAVY   DEEP SEA BLUE   TEAL   MIDNIGHT BLUE

Violet

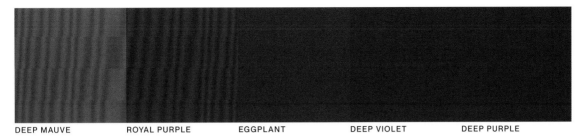

DEEP MAUVE   ROYAL PURPLE   EGGPLANT   DEEP VIOLET   DEEP PURPLE

Neutrals

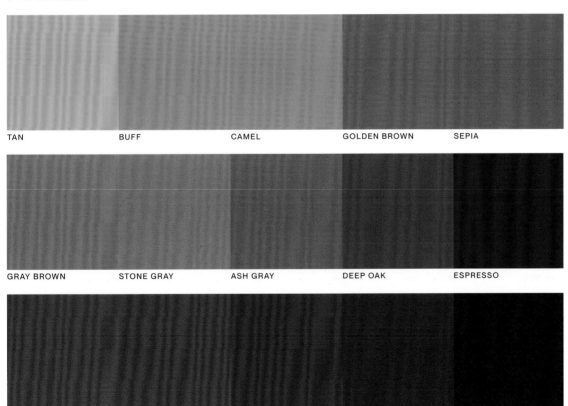

TAN   BUFF   CAMEL   GOLDEN BROWN   SEPIA

GRAY BROWN   STONE GRAY   ASH GRAY   DEEP OAK   ESPRESSO

WALNUT   CHESTNUT   WARM BROWN   RUSSET   MAHOGANY

DEEP WINTER

Color essence Brilliant and intense
Best colors Cool-neutral Rich Shades and Jewel Tones

Deep Winters are characterized by your striking deep features and overall intensity. Just like all Winter types, your coloring is cool-toned and high-contrast. But your medium chroma puts you on the verge of the Autumn season, adding a touch of earthy richness to your color essence.

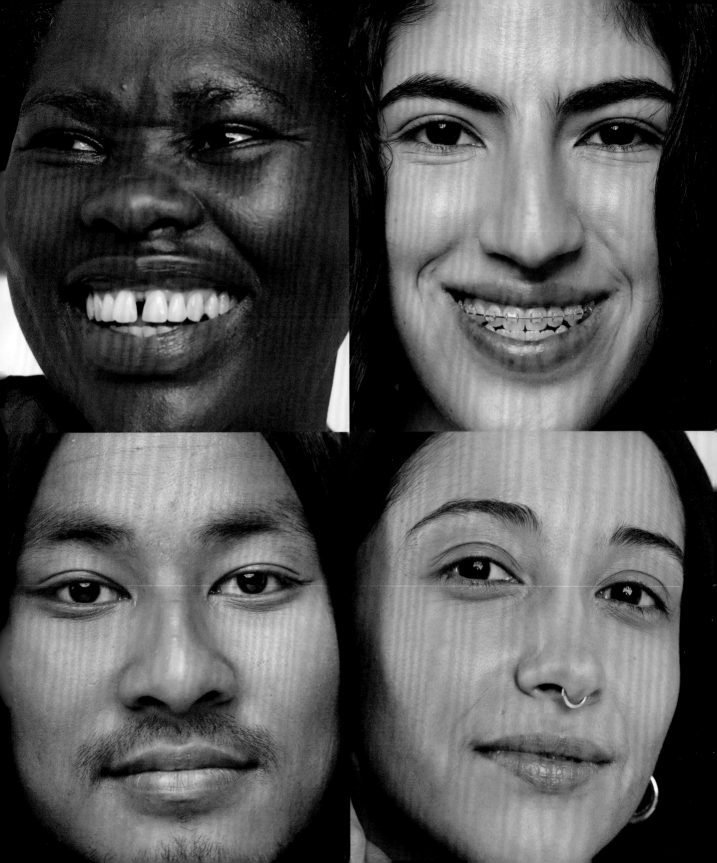

Your best colors

Like all Winters, you look amazing in Jewel Tones. Due to your medium chroma, Rich Shades are also a perfect fit for your coloring.

Across all color genres, cool-neutral shades best harmonize with your undertone. This is a selection of colors that would be perfect for you:

Cool-neutral Rich Shades

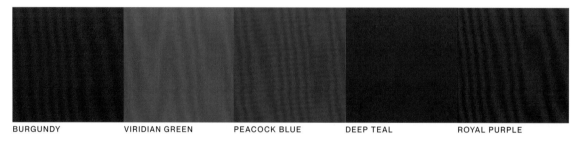

| BURGUNDY | VIRIDIAN GREEN | PEACOCK BLUE | DEEP TEAL | ROYAL PURPLE |

Cool-neutral Jewel Tones

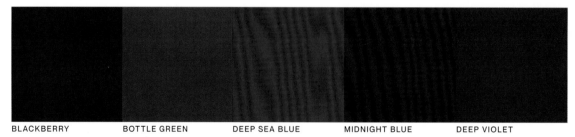

| BLACKBERRY | BOTTLE GREEN | DEEP SEA BLUE | MIDNIGHT BLUE | DEEP VIOLET |

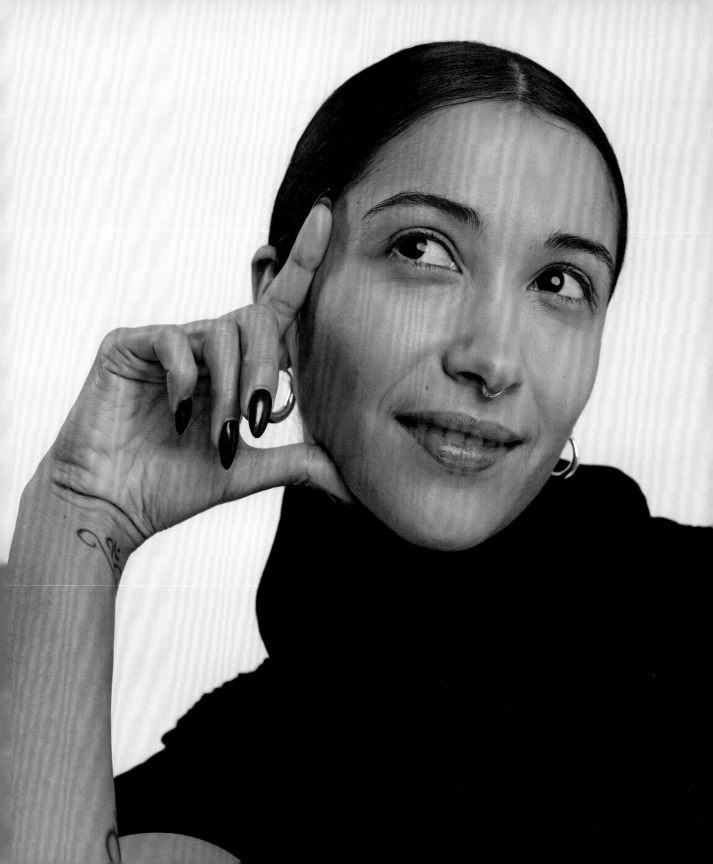

Levels of harmony

The best colors for Deep Winters are cool-neutral Rich Shades and Jewel Tones. Dusky Shades and Vivids will also look good, though they won't be a perfect match. Deep Winter is a cool-neutral season, meaning your palette consists mainly of cool-neutral and cool shades. You will also see some warm-neutral shades (in your best color genres only). Warm shades are not a part of the Deep Winter palette.

Here is an overview of how well different undertones and color genres work on Deep Winters. Ratings for color genres are based on shades that match your best undertone (cool-neutral). Shades in other undertones will be less harmonious.

	Color genre	Undertone
PERFECT MATCH	Jewel Tones Rich Shades	Cool-neutral
HARMONIOUS	Vivids Dusky Shades	Cool
OKAY	Brights	Warm-neutral
DISSONANT	Moderates Pastels	Warm
CLASH	Pale Tones Dimmed Tones	

Your "opposite" colors

Warm Pale Tones and Dimmed Tones are your least harmonious colors. They don't echo any aspect of your coloring, and may clash with your complexion. Here are some examples:

Warm Pale Tones

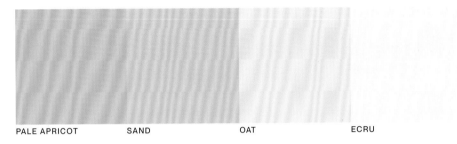

PALE APRICOT   SAND   OAT   ECRU

Warm Dimmed Tones

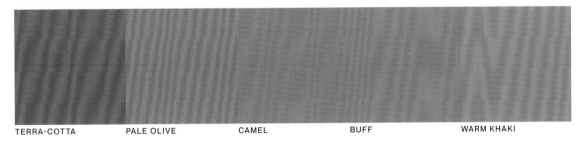

TERRA-COTTA   PALE OLIVE   CAMEL   BUFF   WARM KHAKI

How aging may affect your best colors

Like all seasons, Deep Winters lose some of their chroma and contrast with age. This means that the Vivids and Jewel Tones in your palette may start to look slightly less harmonious, while Dusky Shades may become more harmonious. The undertone of your best colors will remain stable throughout your life.

How a suntan may affect your best colors

If your skin tone is fair or light, a strong suntan will warm up your complexion. As a result, warm-neutral hues will likely be harmonious instead of okay. Regardless of your skin tone, a strong suntan will also increase your chroma somewhat, allowing you to pull off Brights.

Best colors by hue

This section will look at your full color palette, broken down by hue. Note that we will cover hair colors, makeup, and jewelry in later chapters!

Red and pink

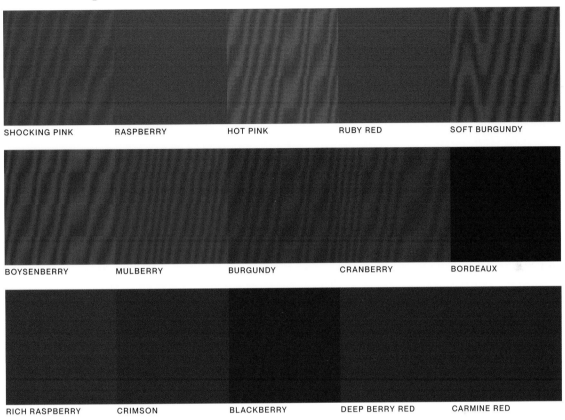

SHOCKING PINK   RASPBERRY   HOT PINK   RUBY RED   SOFT BURGUNDY

BOYSENBERRY   MULBERRY   BURGUNDY   CRANBERRY   BORDEAUX

RICH RASPBERRY   CRIMSON   BLACKBERRY   DEEP BERRY RED   CARMINE RED

Green

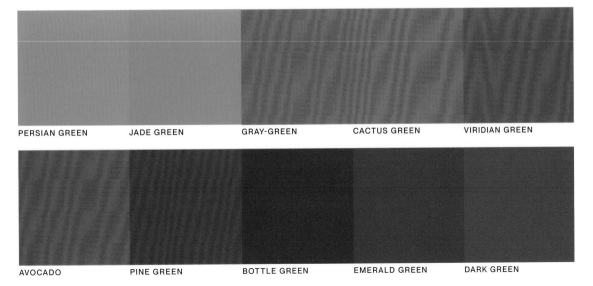

PERSIAN GREEN   JADE GREEN   GRAY-GREEN   CACTUS GREEN   VIRIDIAN GREEN

AVOCADO   PINE GREEN   BOTTLE GREEN   EMERALD GREEN   DARK GREEN

Cyan and blue

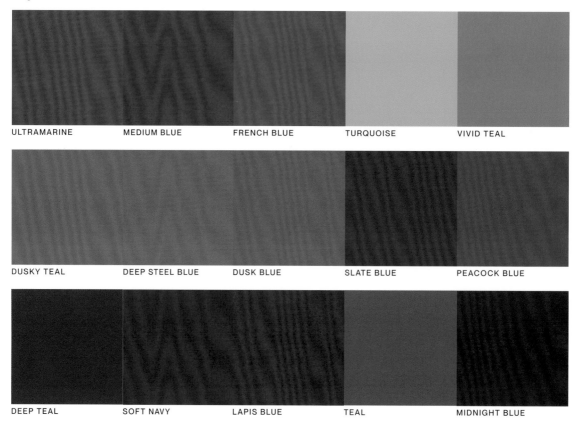

| ULTRAMARINE | MEDIUM BLUE | FRENCH BLUE | TURQUOISE | VIVID TEAL |

| DUSKY TEAL | DEEP STEEL BLUE | DUSK BLUE | SLATE BLUE | PEACOCK BLUE |

| DEEP TEAL | SOFT NAVY | LAPIS BLUE | TEAL | MIDNIGHT BLUE |

Violet

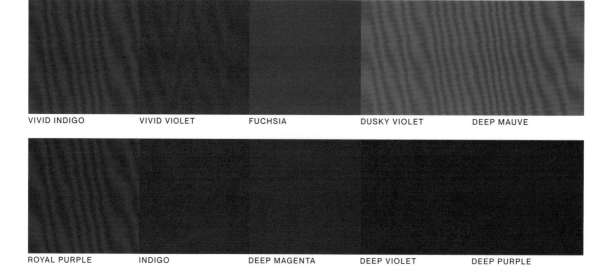

| VIVID INDIGO | VIVID VIOLET | FUCHSIA | DUSKY VIOLET | DEEP MAUVE |

| ROYAL PURPLE | INDIGO | DEEP MAGENTA | DEEP VIOLET | DEEP PURPLE |

Neutrals

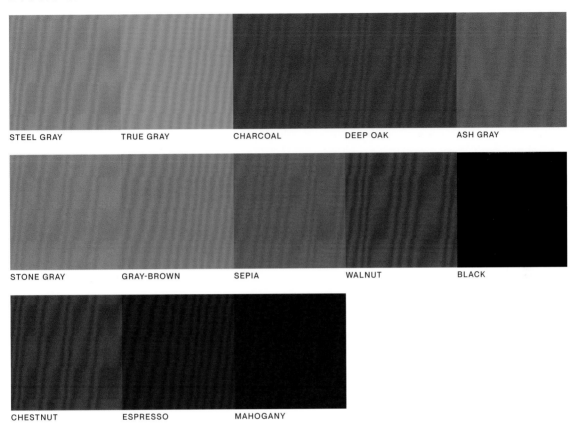

STEEL GRAY TRUE GRAY CHARCOAL DEEP OAK ASH GRAY

STONE GRAY GRAY-BROWN SEPIA WALNUT BLACK

CHESTNUT ESPRESSO MAHOGANY

TRUE WINTER

Color essence Cool and brilliant

Best colors Cool Brights, Vivids, and Jewel Tones

True Winters are the epitome of icy brilliance. Your coloring is clear, high-contrast, and obviously cool. You naturally possess a ton of vibrance and can pull off both monochrome shades and bold, bright colors, as long as they are obviously cool-toned.

Your high contrast level allows you to pull off the full value spectrum: from the iciest shades to the deepest almost-blacks. True Winter is the only season that looks good in white and black.

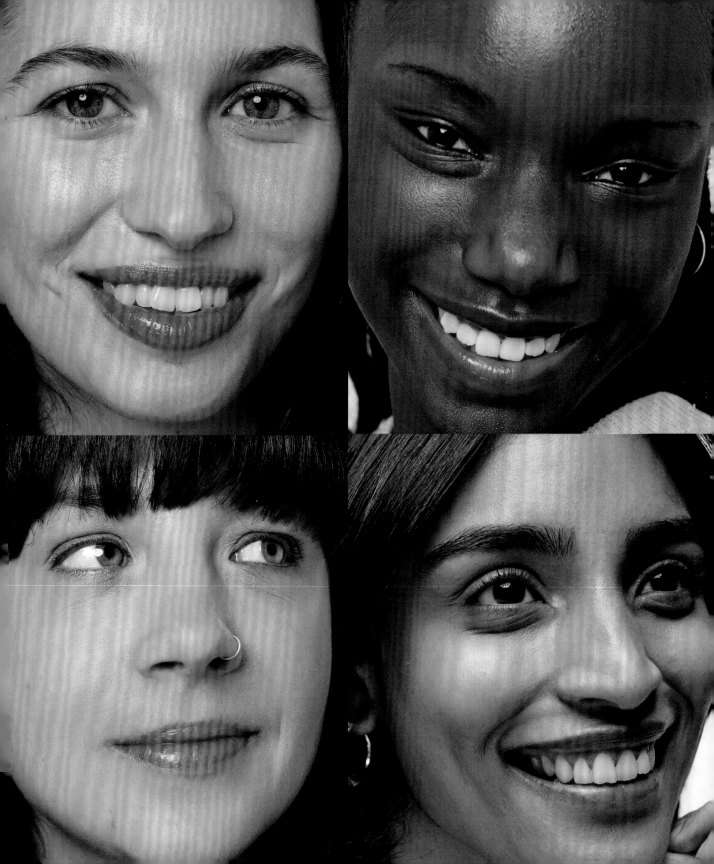

Your best colors

All three high-chroma genres echo your coloring: Brights, Vivids, and Jewel Tones. Across all color genres, shades with a pronounced cool undertone work best.

Let's look at some of your very best colors:

Cool Brights

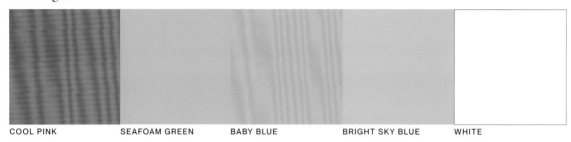

| COOL PINK | SEAFOAM GREEN | BABY BLUE | BRIGHT SKY BLUE | WHITE |

Cool Vivids

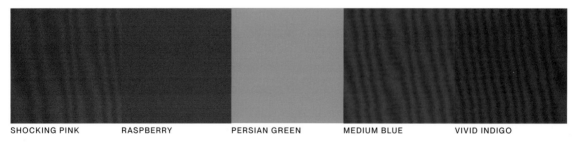

| SHOCKING PINK | RASPBERRY | PERSIAN GREEN | MEDIUM BLUE | VIVID INDIGO |

Cool Jewel Tones

| RICH RASPBERRY | DEEP MAGENTA | LAPIS BLUE | MIDNIGHT BLUE | INDIGO |

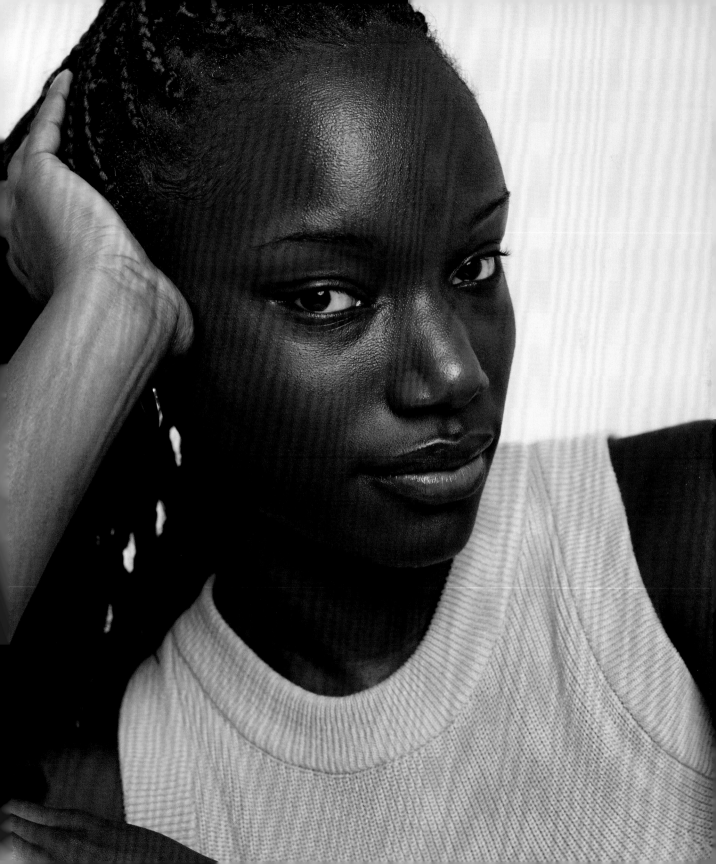

Levels of harmony

True Winters shine in cool Brights, Vivids, and Jewel Tones, but several other color genres will also look reasonably harmonious. Rich Shades (including pure black) are a tad too desaturated to be a perfect match, but they will still look good on you and far from dissonant. As a true cool season, you are less flexible when it comes to the undertone of your shades. Any bit of warmth is likely going to look dissonant on your complexion, which is why your palette consists of exclusively cool and cool-neutral shades. Consequently, you won't find any orange hues in your palette, and your selection of brown neutrals is sparse.

Here is an overview of how well different undertones and color genres work on True Winters. Ratings for color genres are based

	Color genre	Undertone
PERFECT MATCH	Jewel Tones Vivids Brights	Cool
HARMONIOUS	Rich Shades	Cool-neutral
OKAY	Moderates	
DISSONANT	Pastels Dusky Shades	Warm-neutral
CLASH	Dimmed Tones Pale Tones	Warm

on shades that match your best undertone (cool). Shades in other undertones will be less harmonious.

Your "opposite" colors

Warm Pale Tones and Dimmed Tones are your least harmonious colors. They don't echo any aspect of your coloring, and may clash with your complexion. Here are some examples:

Warm Pale Tones

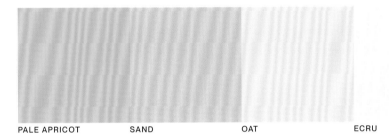

PALE APRICOT   SAND   OAT   ECRU

Warm Dimmed Tones

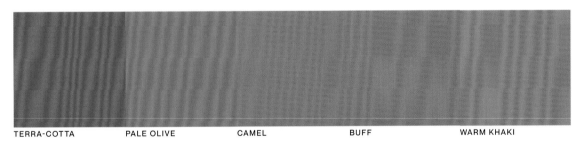

TERRA-COTTA   PALE OLIVE   CAMEL   BUFF   WARM KHAKI

How aging may affect your best colors

Like all seasons, True Winters lose some of their chroma and contrast with age. This means that the Jewel Tones and Brights in your palette may start to look slightly less harmonious, while Rich Shades may become more harmonious. The undertone of your best colors will remain stable throughout your life.

How a suntan may affect your best colors

If your skin tone is fair or light, a strong suntan will warm up your complexion. As a result, warm-neutral hues will likely appear okay instead of dissonant. Regardless of your skin tone, a strong suntan will increase your chroma somewhat, allowing you to pull off fluorescent, neon colors.

Best colors by hue

In this section, we will take a look at your full color palette, broken down by hue. Note that we will cover hair colors, makeup, and jewelry in later chapters!

Red and pink

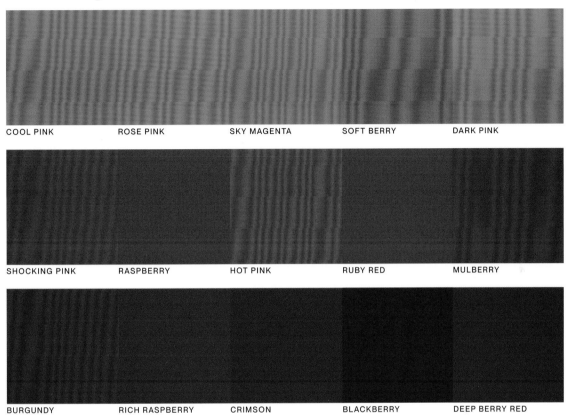

COOL PINK   ROSE PINK   SKY MAGENTA   SOFT BERRY   DARK PINK

SHOCKING PINK   RASPBERRY   HOT PINK   RUBY RED   MULBERRY

BURGUNDY   RICH RASPBERRY   CRIMSON   BLACKBERRY   DEEP BERRY RED

Green

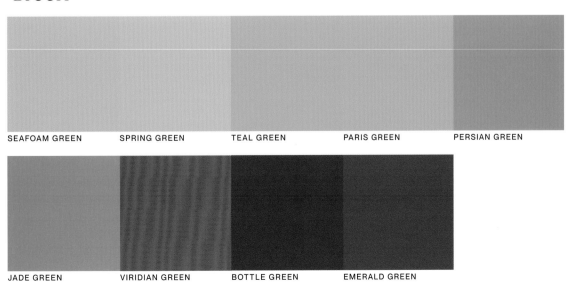

SEAFOAM GREEN   SPRING GREEN   TEAL GREEN   PARIS GREEN   PERSIAN GREEN

JADE GREEN   VIRIDIAN GREEN   BOTTLE GREEN   EMERALD GREEN

Cyan and blue

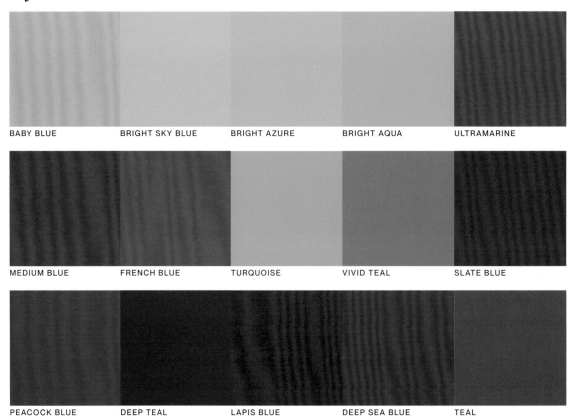

BABY BLUE	BRIGHT SKY BLUE	BRIGHT AZURE	BRIGHT AQUA	ULTRAMARINE
MEDIUM BLUE	FRENCH BLUE	TURQUOISE	VIVID TEAL	SLATE BLUE
PEACOCK BLUE	DEEP TEAL	LAPIS BLUE	DEEP SEA BLUE	TEAL

Violet

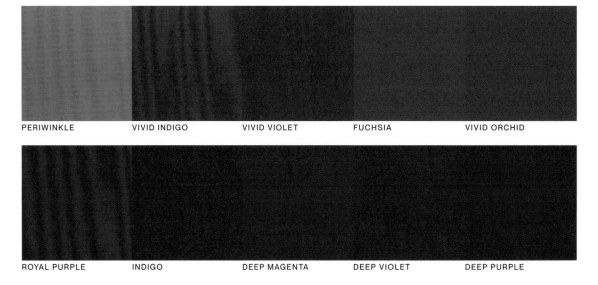

| PERIWINKLE | VIVID INDIGO | VIVID VIOLET | FUCHSIA | VIVID ORCHID |
| ROYAL PURPLE | INDIGO | DEEP MAGENTA | DEEP VIOLET | DEEP PURPLE |

Neutrals

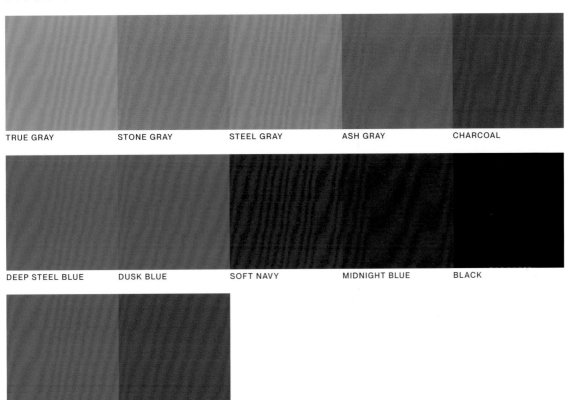

TRUE GRAY   STONE GRAY   STEEL GRAY   ASH GRAY   CHARCOAL

DEEP STEEL BLUE   DUSK BLUE   SOFT NAVY   MIDNIGHT BLUE   BLACK

SEPIA   DEEP OAK

CLEAR WINTER

Color essence Brilliant and luminous
Best colors Cool-neutral Brights,
Vivids, and Jewel Tones

Like all Winter seasons, your coloring is clear and cool, but you also have a bit of Spring in you! Your season is terribly misunderstood: contrary to popular belief, Clear Winters are not simply Winter types with an extremely high chroma. Clear Winters also have considerably lower contrast than other Winters, and do not appear obviously cool. This moderate intensity paired with a clear chroma and almost-neutral undertone is what characterizes this season.

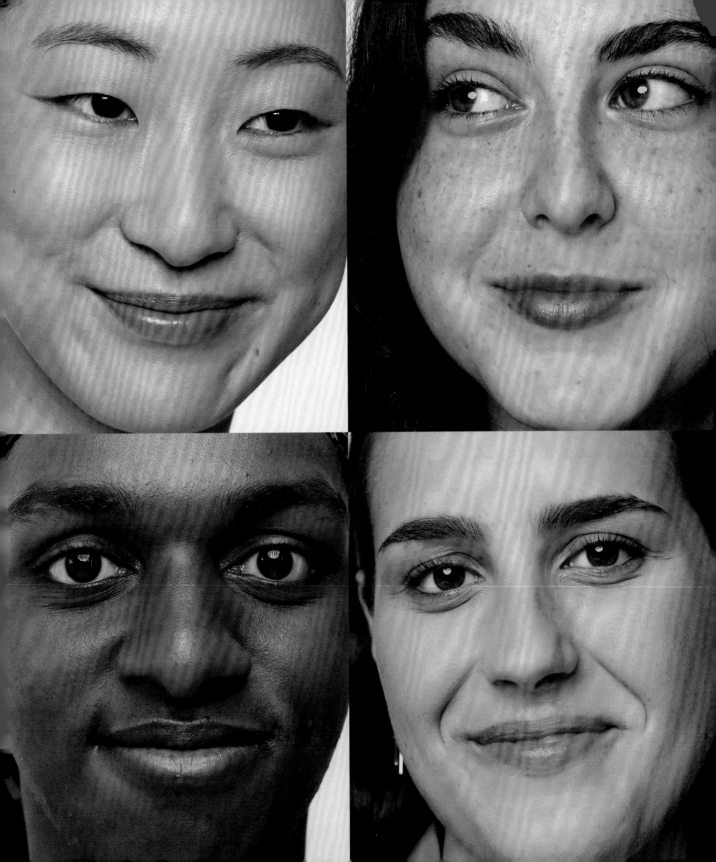

Your best colors

As a Clear Winter, you will struggle finding a color that is too vibrant for you. All of your best colors are highly saturated: Brights, Vivids, and Jewel Tones. You are the only Winter type who does not do well with very deep or very light shades, because they don't contain the chroma you need.

Regardless of color genre, cool-neutral shades best echo your own undertone. Here are some of your best colors:

Cool-neutral Brights

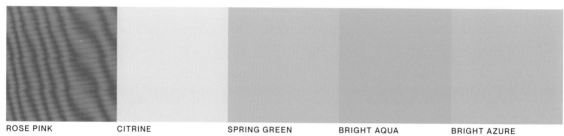

ROSE PINK   CITRINE   SPRING GREEN   BRIGHT AQUA   BRIGHT AZURE

Cool-neutral Vivids

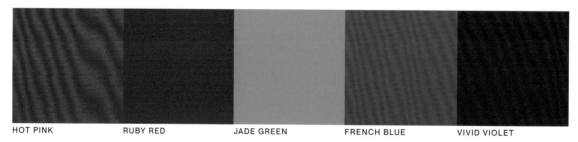

HOT PINK   RUBY RED   JADE GREEN   FRENCH BLUE   VIVID VIOLET

Cool-neutral Jewel Tones

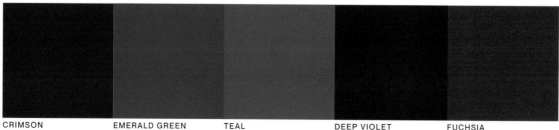

CRIMSON   EMERALD GREEN   TEAL   DEEP VIOLET   FUCHSIA

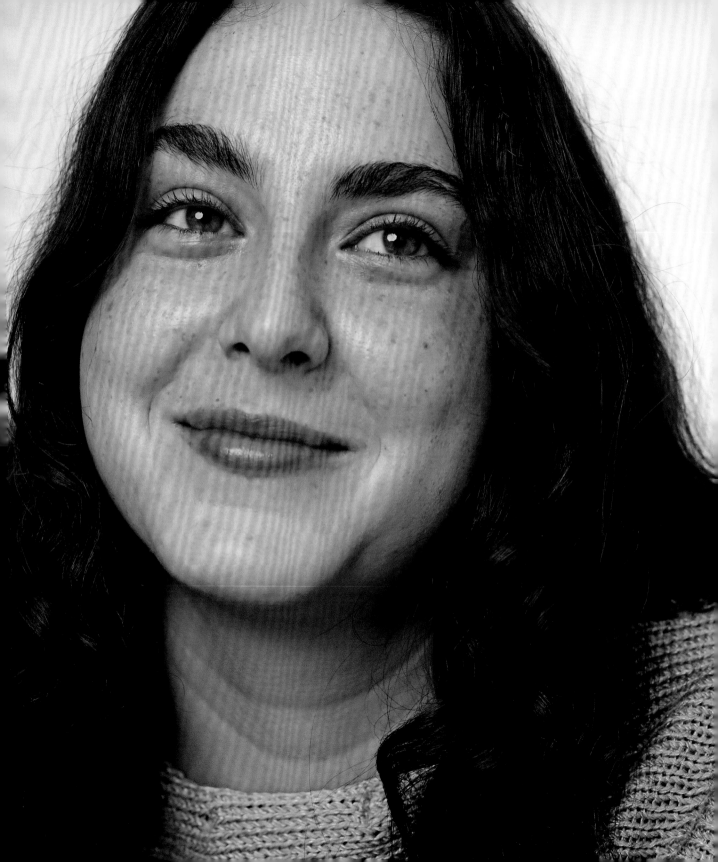

Levels of harmony

Your high chroma and moderate coloring makes you extremely versatile. While cool-neutral Brights, Vivids, and Jewel Tones best honor your color essence, Rich Shades will look almost as harmonious. And while the Clear Winter palette features mostly cool-neutral shades, obviously cool shades will also look good. As long as you are wearing your best color genres, warm-neutral shades also won't clash with your complexion. Only warm shades are not a part of the Clear Winter palette.

Here is an overview of how well different undertones and color genres work on Clear Winters. Ratings for color genres are based on shades that match your best undertone (cool-neutral). Shades in other undertones will be less harmonious.

	Color genre	Undertone
PERFECT MATCH	Vivids Jewel Tones Brights	Cool-neutral
HARMONIOUS	Rich Shades	Cool
OKAY	Moderates	Warm-neutral
DISSONANT	Dusky Shades Pastels	Warm
CLASH	Dimmed Tones Pale Tones	

Your "opposite" colors

Warm Pale Tones and Dimmed Tones are your least harmonious colors. They don't echo any aspect of your coloring, and may clash with your complexion. Here are some examples:

Warm Pale Tones

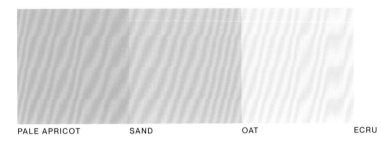

PALE APRICOT   SAND   OAT   ECRU

Warm Dimmed Tones

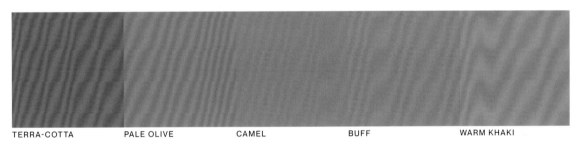

TERRA-COTTA   PALE OLIVE   CAMEL   BUFF   WARM KHAKI

How aging may affect your best colors

Like all seasons, Clear Winters lose some of their chroma and contrast with age. This means that the Brights and Jewel Tones in your palette may start to look slightly less harmonious, while Moderates and Pastels may become more harmonious. The undertone of your best colors will remain stable throughout your life.

How a suntan may affect your best colors

If your skin tone is fair or light, a strong suntan will warm up your complexion. As a result, warm-neutral hues will likely be harmonious instead of okay. Regardless of your skin tone, a strong suntan will increase your chroma somewhat, allowing you to pull off fluorescent, neon colors.

Best colors by hue

In this section, we will take a look at your full color palette, broken down by hue. Note that we will cover hair colors, makeup, and jewelry in later chapters!

Red and pink

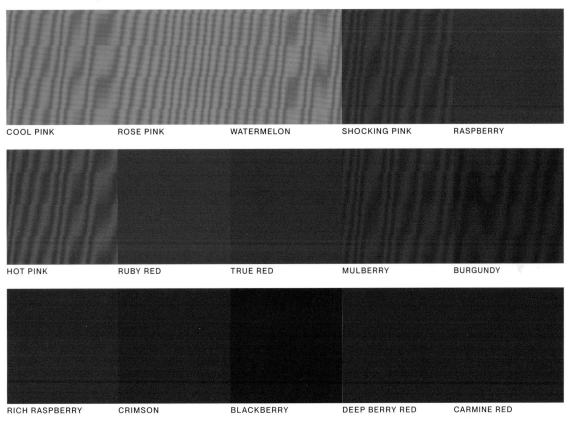

COOL PINK	ROSE PINK	WATERMELON	SHOCKING PINK	RASPBERRY
HOT PINK	RUBY RED	TRUE RED	MULBERRY	BURGUNDY
RICH RASPBERRY	CRIMSON	BLACKBERRY	DEEP BERRY RED	CARMINE RED

Orange and yellow

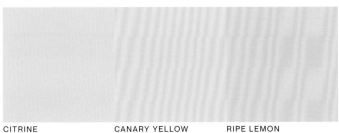

CITRINE   CANARY YELLOW   RIPE LEMON

Green

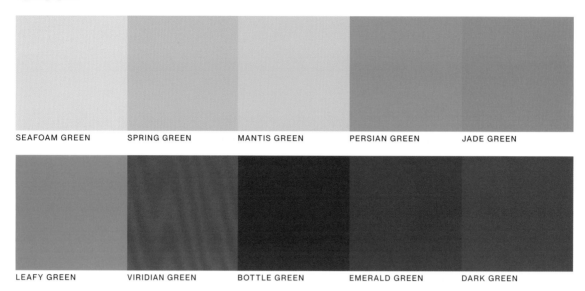

SEAFOAM GREEN   SPRING GREEN   MANTIS GREEN   PERSIAN GREEN   JADE GREEN

LEAFY GREEN   VIRIDIAN GREEN   BOTTLE GREEN   EMERALD GREEN   DARK GREEN

Cyan and blue

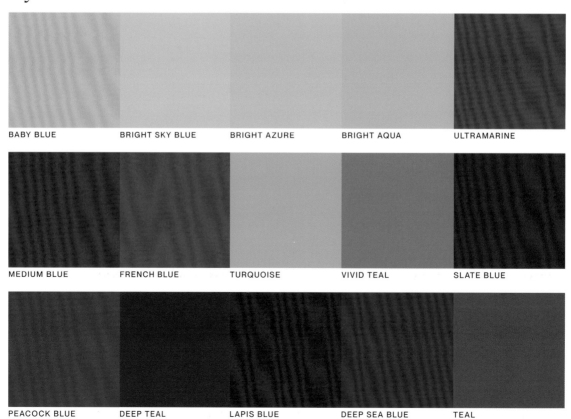

BABY BLUE   BRIGHT SKY BLUE   BRIGHT AZURE   BRIGHT AQUA   ULTRAMARINE

MEDIUM BLUE   FRENCH BLUE   TURQUOISE   VIVID TEAL   SLATE BLUE

PEACOCK BLUE   DEEP TEAL   LAPIS BLUE   DEEP SEA BLUE   TEAL

Violet

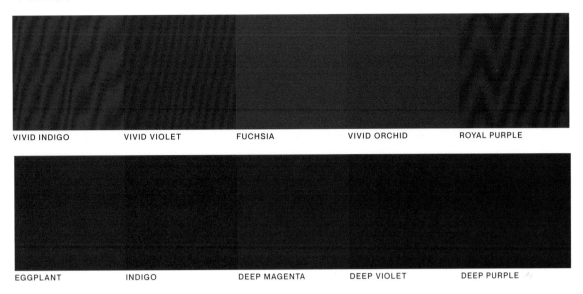

VIVID INDIGO	VIVID VIOLET	FUCHSIA	VIVID ORCHID	ROYAL PURPLE
EGGPLANT	INDIGO	DEEP MAGENTA	DEEP VIOLET	DEEP PURPLE

Neutrals

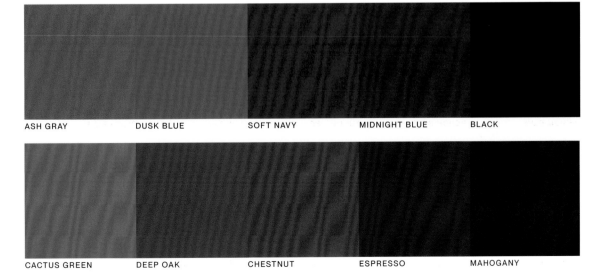

ASH GRAY	DUSK BLUE	SOFT NAVY	MIDNIGHT BLUE	BLACK
CACTUS GREEN	DEEP OAK	CHESTNUT	ESPRESSO	MAHOGANY

GOLD OR SILVER

What Color Jewelry Works Best for Your Season?

You've probably heard that cool undertones look better in silver jewelry and warm undertones look better in gold jewelry, but actually, it's not that simple . . .

If you put two random pieces of gold jewelry side by side, chances are they will look quite different. One gold may be saturated and warm; the other may be softer and cooler. The same goes for silver jewelry: One piece may have a bright, platinum tone, while another is a darker, blue-tinged gray.

Those are pretty significant differences in undertone, chroma, and value. So, the question is not "Does silver or gold work best with my coloring?" but rather "Which shade of silver and which shade of gold works best?"

Before we get into the world of gold, silver, and all their variations, let's remember the two rules of color impact: proximity to your face and scale. While some jewelry might be near your face, most pieces are just too small to have a big impact on your overall look. Of course, big statement necklaces and earrings are a different story. But there is no need to overthink every dainty necklace or stop wearing pieces you love for the sake of color harmony.

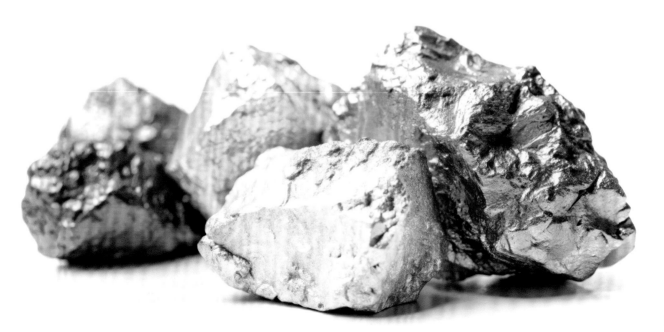

Shades of gold

Pure fine gold has a bright yellow color that is very warm and saturated. But gold jewelry is rarely made of 100 percent pure gold because it's too soft. Instead, jewelers melt the gold and mix in a certain portion of other precious metals, usually silver or copper. The resulting mixture is called an alloy. The shade of a piece of gold jewelry depends on the exact components of its alloy.

Silver has a bright, light gray tone; it is a true grayscale shade, without any sort of chroma. Mixing silver into a gold alloy desaturates and lightens the color. Copper has a saturated orange-red tone. Fine gold has a warmer undertone than raw copper, so the more copper that is added to fine gold, the cooler the gold alloy will be. Of course, it won't be cool in absolute terms—this is still an orange hue that we are talking about.

Only fine gold jewelry consists of solid gold alloy. Gold-filled or gold-plated pieces consist of a brass or steel core that has been coated in a thin layer of fine gold alloy. Since the fine gold coating is what determines the shade of a gold-filled or gold-plated piece, all the same information applies.

Depending on how much copper or silver is added to the gold alloy, gold jewelry will have one of the following shades.

Warm yellow gold

Warm yellow gold comes closest to the shade of pure gold. This shade of gold can be found in higher karat gold jewelry, as these pieces will have fewer other metals mixed into the alloy.

As a color genre, warm yellow gold is a Vivid with a warm undertone. It's a perfect match for Clear Springs, True Springs, and True Autumns, and will also work well on all other Autumn and Spring seasons.

Pale yellow gold

When the gold alloy contains a larger amount of silver, the resulting color will be a pale, desaturated yellow.

Pale yellow gold is a warm-neutral Pale Tone. As such, it works well on Soft Autumns, True Springs, and Light Springs, and it looks good on all other Autumn and Spring seasons, as well as Light Summers.

What is white gold?

White gold is meant to mimic the bright shade of platinum. It is usually created by coating yellow gold with a thin plating of rhodium (another silvery-white precious metal). Although white gold is physically gold, its color properties are those of silver.

Apricot gold

A peachy yellow gold, this shade is halfway to being a rose gold, with a relatively high copper content. Apricot gold is a warm-neutral Pastel, which makes it a perfect match for all Spring types and also tends to work well on Light Summers.

Deep yellow gold

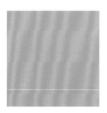

A deeper yellow with a slight greenish tinge is common in fine gold pieces at lower karats (or in gold-plated pieces). Because of its deeper value, deep yellow gold is a warm-neutral Rich Shade, making it an ideal match for all Autumn seasons, and also suitable for Deep Winters.

Rose gold

When fine gold is mixed with a large amount of copper, we get rose gold, which used to be called red gold. Rose gold is a warm-neutral Pastel that is almost neutral in undertone, making it the most universally flattering gold shade.

Shades of silver

Silver jewelry varies less in tone than gold jewelry because silver alloy usually has a smaller amount of other metals mixed in. But some of what is sold as silver-colored jewelry is not actually silver but stainless steel, which is considerably deeper and cooler. Here is how to differentiate among types of silver-colored jewelry.

Sterling silver

Just like fine gold, fine silver needs a touch of copper to be strong enough to work as jewelry. A popular alloy is sterling silver, comprising 92.5 percent silver and 7.5 percent copper. The tone of sterling silver is generally consistent and not much different from pure silver: It's very light in value and cool-neutral in undertone. The same goes for silver-filled and silver-plated jewelry, which consists of a brass or steel core coated in the same sterling silver alloy.

Due to its reflective properties, sterling silver comes closest to a cool-neutral Bright, making it an ideal match for Light Summers, True Winters, and Clear Winters, and a better match than gold for all other Summer and Winter types.

Stainless steel

Silver and steel have pretty different color properties. Steel is darker and quite a bit cooler than silver, and it often has a noticeable green or blue tint, making it closest to a cool Dimmed Tone. As such, stainless steel jewelry will work better than silver on Soft Summers, Deep Winters, and all Autumn types. In contrast, stainless steel is less harmonious than silver on Light Summers, Clear Winters, and all Spring types. True Summers and True Winters will do equally well with both.

Oxidized silver

Oxidized silver is sterling silver processed to develop a deep patina that gives it an antique finish. The result is often a sort of anthracite shade that can be pretty deep. Like other cool-toned Dusky Shades, oxidized silver perfectly matches only Soft Summers and Deep Winters. To a lesser degree, it will also harmonize with True Summers, Soft Autumns, Deep Autumns, and True Winters.

	Warm Yellow Gold	Pale Yellow Gold	Deep Yellow Gold	Apricot Gold	Rose Gold	Sterling Silver	Stainless Steel	Oxidized Silver
SPRING								
Clear	●	●	●	●	●	●	●	●
True	●	●	●	●	●	●	●	●
Light	●	●	●	●	●	●	●	●
SUMMER								
Light	●	●	●	●	●	●	●	●
True	●	●	●	●	●	●	●	●
Soft	●	●	●	●	●	●	●	●
AUTUMN								
Soft	●	●	●	●	●	●	●	●
True	●	●	●	●	●	●	●	●
Deep	●	●	●	●	●	●	●	●
WINTER								
Deep	●	●	●	●	●	●	●	●
True	●	●	●	●	●	●	●	●
Clear	●	●	●	●	●	●	●	●

● Perfect match
● Harmonious
● Okay
● Dissonant
● Clash

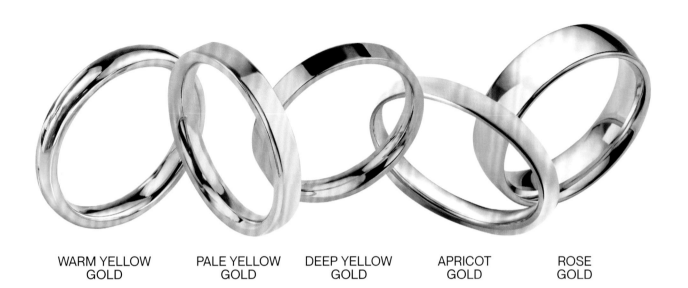

WARM YELLOW
GOLD

PALE YELLOW
GOLD

DEEP YELLOW
GOLD

APRICOT
GOLD

ROSE
GOLD

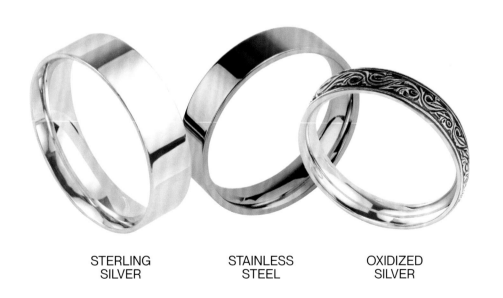

STERLING
SILVER

STAINLESS
STEEL

OXIDIZED
SILVER

HAIR
COLOR

How to Find the Right Hair
Level and Tone for Your Season

If there is only one thing you align to your season, make it your hair color. Since it is so close to your face, finding a shade that truly complements your color essence can be transformative. On the other hand, a less harmonious hue can throw off your whole look, clash with your skin tone, and add shadows where there are none. If your strands have never been touched by bleach, dye, or toner, you've already won the color harmony game. Your natural shade will always complement your coloring (that includes hair that has entirely gone gray). But what if you want to switch things up? What if your hair is toffee brown, but you're in the mood for a touch of red? Or maybe you've always wanted to go darker and try a rich espresso shade? Or add some dimension with caramel highlights? How about an icy silver? The options are endless, and the good news is that your natural color—while always a good match for your season—is not your best or only match.

No matter your season and skin tone, a variety of shades can help you embrace your unique color essence. In this chapter, we'll explore all of your options and equip you with the terminology you need to communicate your color preferences effectively to a hair professional.

Hair level and tone

All of your best hair colors will be two things: the right level and the right tone for your coloring.

Hair level and tone are concepts used by hairstylists and colorists worldwide to classify hair colors.

You already know from page 88 that hair level refers to the base color of a shade, ranging from 1 to 10 (black to the lightest blond). There is also a level 10+, which is an almost-white shade that forms the basis for colors like platinum blond or an icy gray.

Hair tone refers to the hue of a shade (beyond its base color). Common tones are blue, purple, mahogany (a mix of purple and red), red, copper, and gold, but any hue on the spectrum could serve as a hair tone.

Every hair color is a combination of a hair level with a specific hair tone. For example, a mahogany tone on level 4 hair will create a deep auburn shade. A blue tone on level 6 hair results in an ashy mushroom brown. A gold tone on level 8 hair creates a warm honey blond. In this chapter, we'll figure out your ideal hair levels and tones separately. You will likely end up with a range of hair levels and several hair tones that all harmonize with your coloring—for example, hair levels 6 to 8, and blue, purple, and mahogany tones. Then, we'll explore which hair colors match those levels and tones.

A note on the term *undertone*

Hair and beauty professionals tend to use the term *undertone* in a different way than it is used in color theory. It's good to keep this difference in mind to avoid any confusion when you are looking for color inspiration online or discussing shade options at the salon.

In color theory, *undertone* refers to the temperature of a shade, from cool to warm. Any hue can have any undertone, and a shade's undertone is relative to its hue family. Undertones can either be warm or cool.

In the hair and beauty industry, the term *undertone* is often used to indicate that the main shade contains small amounts of another shade. For instance, a hair professional might describe a silver shade as having purple undertones, which means that the shade is primarily silver, but with a subtle tint of purple mixed in. Or they may say that a particular red has brown undertones, to refer to a shade that is predominantly red but leans toward a brown hue on the color wheel.

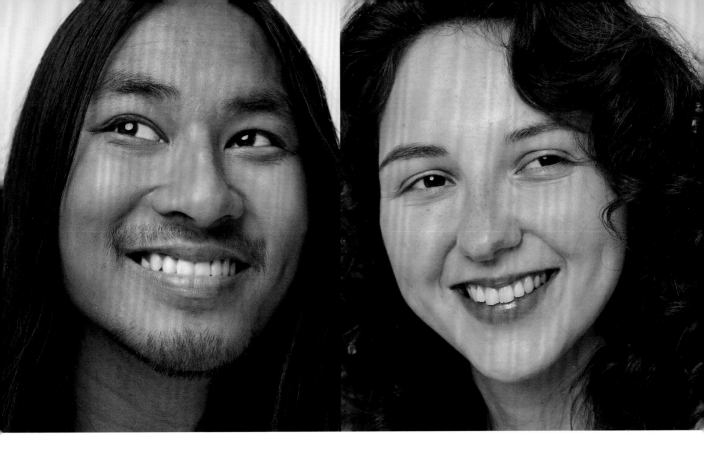

Hair level: How deep or light should your hair be?

The ideal hair level for your coloring will honor your overall contrast level: Too little contrast may make you look washed out, like your features lack definition, while too much contrast may overwhelm your coloring, appear stark, and emphasize shadows on your face.

Your contrast level tells you how much deeper or lighter than your skin tone your hair should be.

Contrast level

VERY HIGH	Ideal hair color is much deeper or lighter than skin tone
HIGH	Ideal hair color is considerably deeper or lighter than skin tone
MEDIUM	Ideal hair color is somewhat deeper or lighter than skin tone
LOW	Ideal hair color is not much deeper or lighter than skin tone

As a rule of thumb, any hair color that is roughly as deep as your natural hair color will always create an optimal amount of contrast against your skin tone. But a range of hair levels will create the contrast you need, and you may be able to go quite a bit lighter or deeper than your natural hair color.

For example, let's say you have a light-medium skin tone and your natural hair color is a level 4 dark brown. Multiple hair levels will help you echo your medium contrast level—going darker to a level 3 would give you too much contrast, but going lighter to a level 5 would retain your medium contrast. Anything lighter than that is too low-contrast (i.e., too close to your skin tone)—that is, until you get to a 10+ level: A bright platinum blond or white shade is once again different enough from your skin tone to echo your contrast level.

Do not forget that contrast works in both directions! You can create a high contrast level by choosing a hair color that is considerably deeper or lighter than your skin tone. Also, keep in mind that a very high hair level does not have to mean platinum blond. A hair level of 9 to 10+ could be a cool light gray, a pastel pink, or a bright white.

Of course, not all skin tones can go in both directions. If you have fair or light skin, even pure white won't give you more than a low contrast level. But light-medium or medium skin tones with medium contrast levels will look great in very light hair levels (as long as the color fits their undertone, of course). And on deep skin, hair levels 10 and 10+ will create a high contrast level.

Contrast Levels

Hair Level	Skin Tone		Rich-deep	Deep	Medium-deep	Medium	Light-medium	Light	Fair
1	Black		High	High	High	Very high	Very high	Very high	Very high
2	Black-brown		High	High	High	High	Very high	Very high	Very high
3	Darkest brown		Medium	Medium	Medium	High	High	High	Very high
4	Dark brown	Auburn	Low	Medium	Medium	Medium	Medium	High	High
5	Medium brown	Titian	Low	Low	Low	Medium	Medium	Medium	High
6	Light brown	Red	Low	Low	Low	Low	Low	Medium	Medium
7	Dark blond	Copper	Low	Low	Low	Low	Low	Low	Medium
8	Medium blond	Strawberry blond	Medium	Low	Low	Low	Low	Low	Low
9	Light blond	Light strawberry blond	High	Medium	Low	Low	Low	Low	Low
10	Lightest blond	Lightest strawberry blond	High	High	Medium	Medium	Low	Low	Low
10+	Platinum/White		Very high	High	High	Medium	Medium	Low	Low

Which hair tone works for your coloring?

The right hair tone for your coloring echoes your undertone, or at least does not clash with it.

The most common hair tones professional colorists use to dye their clients' hair are:

BLUE   RED

PURPLE   COPPER

MAHOGANY   GOLD

Note that the purpose of blue and purple tones is often not to show up on the hair but to neutralize orange and yellow pigments in the base color, making it cooler and more ashy. Here is an overview of common hair tones and how well they work for each undertone.

	Blue	Purple	Mahogany	Red	Copper	Gold
COOL	Perfect match	Perfect match	Harmonious	Okay	Dissonant	Dissonant
COOL-NEUTRAL	Harmonious	Perfect match	Perfect match	Harmonious	Okay	Okay
WARM-NEUTRAL	Okay	Okay	Harmonious	Perfect match	Perfect match	Harmonious
WARM	Dissonant	Perfect match	Perfect match	Harmonious	Perfect match	Harmonious

Legend:
- ● Perfect match
- ● Harmonious
- ○ Okay
- ● Dissonant
- ● Clash

Hair colors

Now that you know your ideal hair level(s) and hair tones, you can assess how well different hair colors work for your coloring. Note that the stated level of harmony for these is based on proximity to your face. Shades that do not come in visual contact with your face have much less of an impact on color harmony. Also note that any dimension you are adding to your hair in the form of highlights or lowlights may alter the overall level of your shade.

TRUE OR FALSE?
Red hair doesn't work on cool undertones.

False! Most people would probably intuitively say that red hair is harder to pull off than a warm honey blond. But that is not true: Red tones actually work on a broader range of undertones than gold tones. Considering color theory, that makes sense, because true red has a relatively neutral undertone (temperature), while the orange-y hue of gold is very close to peak warmth.

If you are a cool-neutral type, both true reds and purple-y reds will work well, as long as you get the chroma and hair level right.

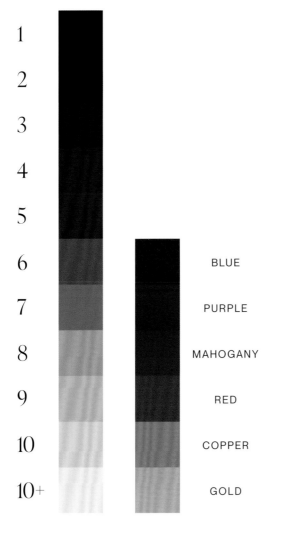

1

2

3

4

5

6   BLUE

7   PURPLE

8   MAHOGANY

9   RED

10   COPPER

10+   GOLD

Cool → Warm

2

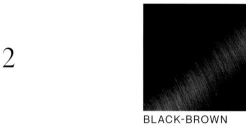

BLACK-BROWN

3

COOL DARKEST BROWN DARKEST BROWN BLACK CHERRY

4

COOL DARK BROWN DARK BROWN AUBURN RICH CHESTNUT

5

COOL MEDIUM BROWN MEDIUM BROWN TITIAN CHOCOLATE BROWN GOLDEN BROWN

6

MUSHROOM BROWN LIGHT BROWN RED WARM LIGHT BROWN TOFFEE

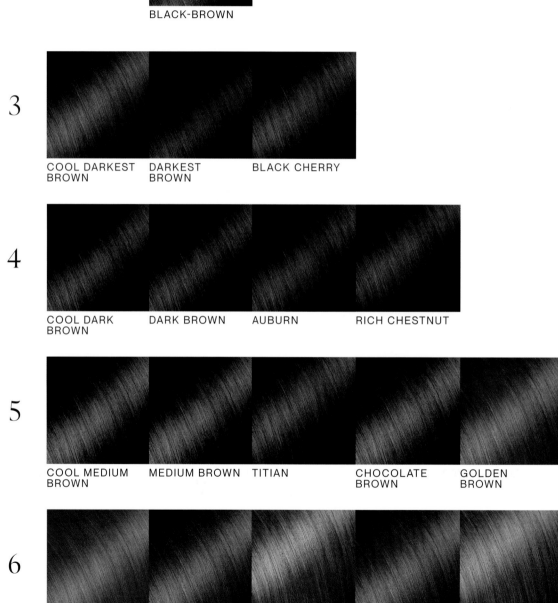

PERSONAL COLOR

316

Cool ← → Warm

7

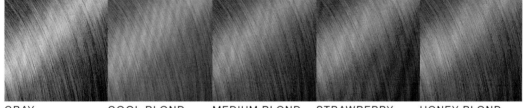

DARK COOL BLOND DARK BLOND COPPER RICH HONEY BLOND

8

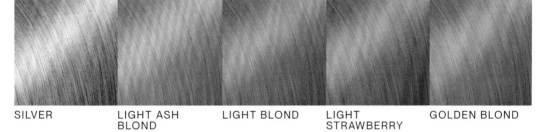

GRAY COOL BLOND MEDIUM BLOND STRAWBERRY BLOND HONEY BLOND

9

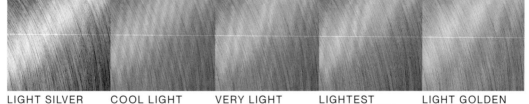

SILVER LIGHT ASH BLOND LIGHT BLOND LIGHT STRAWBERRY BLOND GOLDEN BLOND

10

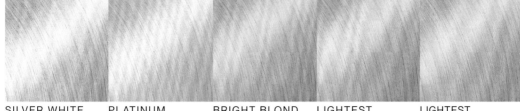

LIGHT SILVER COOL LIGHT BLOND VERY LIGHT BLOND LIGHTEST STRAWBERRY BLOND LIGHT GOLDEN BLOND

10+

SILVER WHITE PLATINUM BLOND BRIGHT BLOND LIGHTEST PEACH LIGHTEST GOLDEN BLOND

MAKEUP

What Works and What Doesn't, for Every Season

When it comes to color harmony, makeup is entirely optional. Regardless of your season, your natural coloring is perfectly harmonious as it is, without a lick of mascara, blush, or concealer. But if you like wearing makeup and it's a form of self-care for you, you absolutely can use it to further lean in to your unique color essence.

Before we explore what type of makeup works for each season, check out the color impact scale below. When it comes to color harmony, some steps in your makeup routine matter a lot more than others. You don't need to worry about every lip gloss, dab of blush, or tiny bit of shimmery shadow you add to the inner corners of your eyes. Nailing the undertone of your base products (like foundation or concealer) is far more important, and we'll discuss exactly how to do that in this chapter. But with makeup, it's not just about which shades you use. It's also about *how* you use them: How much are you applying, how heavy is your hand, how much depth and intensity are you adding to your face? If you want your makeup to look harmonious, you need to know which level of intensity works for your coloring.

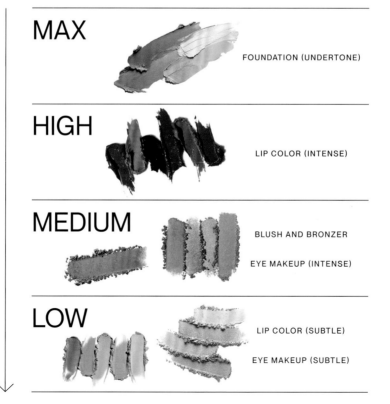

MAX
FOUNDATION (UNDERTONE)

HIGH
LIP COLOR (INTENSE)

MEDIUM
BLUSH AND BRONZER

EYE MAKEUP (INTENSE)

LOW
LIP COLOR (SUBTLE)

EYE MAKEUP (SUBTLE)

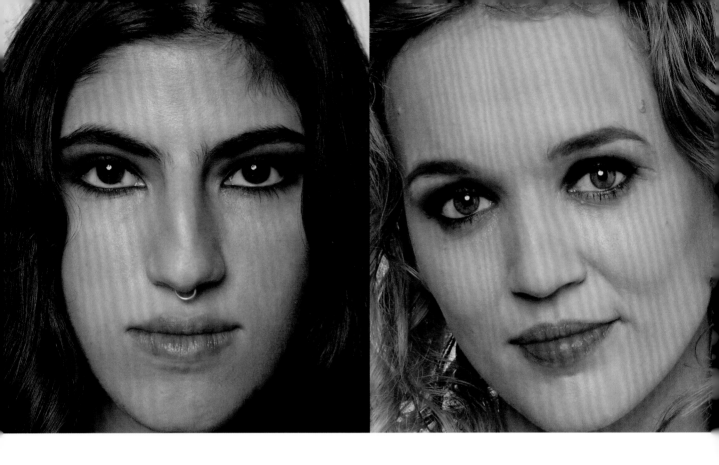

The three rules of intensity

With the same shades, we could create a super-subtle, barely-there look of sheer washes with only hints of color, or a dramatic, all-out statement look. That second look would completely overwhelm one person but look effortless and just right on another.

In the pictures above, Ari (left) and Signe (right) are wearing the same eye makeup. Do you agree that the deep eye shadow feels more dramatic on Signe than on Ari? The critical difference: contrast. Your contrast level is a direct reflection of your capacity for intensity.

There are three important rules for matching the intensity of your makeup to your contrast level.

Intensity rule 1: Adding intensity is always optional

Your natural coloring already has all the contrast it needs for color harmony, so having a high contrast level doesn't mean you should only wear high-intensity makeup. You absolutely could, but you can also wear subtler or no makeup at all. Your coloring is already high contrast; you don't need to add anything if you don't want to. This also goes for low-contrast types, who often feel like their lack of definition is a flaw that needs fixing, when actually it is a key part of what makes their coloring inherently harmonious and unique.

Intensity rule 2: The higher your contrast level, the more intensity you can pull off

Most of us will have a limit when it comes to the amount of intensity we can add before it starts to look jarring. Cross that limit, and your makeup will enter the room before you do.

Very high contrast

You can pull off deep, intense looks like no one else. All-over black, stark graphic liner, rich plum lips, maximum drama: Anyone else would buckle under the weight, but you handle it on a Tuesday. Thanks to all the intensity your coloring naturally possesses, you look effortless and at home in looks that others reserve for special occasions.

High contrast

You are not quite as much of a bottomless pit for makeup as someone with a very high contrast level, but you, too, can handle a lot of makeup. Few looks are too much for you. Your high-contrast coloring can carry off intense definition, deep shades, and bold lip colors.

Medium contrast

As a medium-contrast type, you probably know what it's like to teeter on that line between "just a little more" and "wash it off!" You can handle some definition and some color, but intense depth and bold colors tend to be too much for your complexion.

Low contrast

Your delicate complexion has the lowest capacity for makeup, and even subtle looks can seem harsh on you. That does not mean you can't have fun with makeup! Use a light hand when it comes to anything that adds depth, like mascara, liner, and darker shadows. Opt for transparent, sheer formulas for your lip color and blush.

The three factors that determine the intensity of your makeup

		More intensity	Less intensity
OPACITY	How opaque is the color?	higher coverage products and/or heavier application	sheer, transparent formulas and/or sheer washes of color applied with a lighter hand
DEPTH	How deep are the deepest shades you are using?	deeper shades (compared to your skin tone)	shades that are only slightly deeper than your skin tone
PLACEMENT	How much of your skin are you applying color(s) to?	large area covered in color(s), e.g., entire lid area plus lip	smaller area(s), for example, a thin stroke of eyeliner

Intensity rule 3: Avoid reducing your natural contrast level

While there is no such thing as a minimum amount of makeup, there is a minimum contrast level you need for color harmony, and that is the one you have naturally, so you want to avoid anything that will reduce it. Few things will throw off color harmony more than reducing the amount of contrast you naturally have in your coloring, whether that is a lot or just a little.

"How would I even do that?" you may ask. Besides dying your hair a too-light shade, there are also a few makeup-related things that will reduce your base contrast level:

☐ Lightening or shaving off your eyebrows

☐ Wearing any lip color that is paler than your bare lips

☐ Wearing base makeup that covers the natural blushing and dimension-giving shadows of your face (including around your eyes), without adding color or contour back in

How to match your foundation to your undertone

Picking the right shade for your foundation, concealer, and any other type of base product is critical for color harmony. If you regularly wear makeup, you probably have some experience shopping for a shade that is neither too light nor too dark for your skin. The correct shade won't just match your skin in terms of value, but also in undertone. Honestly, I'd rather you pick a foundation shade that is a little too dark for your skin than one with the wrong undertone. If your skin has a cool undertone, for example, and you apply a warm-toned foundation, not only will your face be a different shade from the rest of your body, but it will also no longer harmonize with the rest of your features.

Fortunately, more and more beauty brands are recognizing the importance of catering to a range of undertones. Of those brands, most distinguish between four undertones:

NEUTRAL   WARM

COOL   OLIVE

Keep in mind that each brand may have a different definition of what constitutes each undertone, which may differ from the definitions we have used in this book. In my experience, the following foundation undertones tend to work best for each skin undertone (but use these recommendations as a starting point only):

☐ Skin with a cool undertone → Cool or neutral foundation (or olive if applicable)

☐ Skin with a cool-neutral undertone → Neutral foundation (or olive if applicable)

☐ Skin with a warm-neutral undertone → Neutral or warm foundation

☐ Skin with a warm undertone → Warm foundation

Why cool foundations don't work on many people

Many cool foundations are formulated for skin with a pink or red tinge, which clashes with our definition of cool skin as simply containing very little orange warmth. In general, cool-neutral skin does better with neutral-toned foundations. There are only two types of skin tones for which a red- or pink-toned foundation is a good choice:

☐ Rich-deep to medium-deep skin tones that are cool-toned due to red pheomelanin (as opposed to a lack of warmth or a yellow tint/olive skin tone).

☐ Fair skin tones that are cool-toned due to a lack of warmth. Skin like this contains very little melanin of any kind, and may appear slightly pink-toned.

Is there an olive undertone?

You already know from page 112 that olive is not actually an undertone but the result of yellow pheomelanin and that most people with olive skin have a cool undertone. But since olive skin can differ in hue from non-olive cool skin tones, it makes sense to offer separate shades. Most olive foundation shades seem to cater to cool-toned olives. If your undertone is warm, those foundations may make your skin look a touch gray.

Lip colors

The next page features a selection of lip color options for every season. Keep in mind that you still need to make sure you are applying the shades at a level of intensity that works for your contrast level. The sheerer the color, the lower the intensity. The deeper the shade compared to your skin tone, the higher the intensity. And regardless of the opacity or depth of your lip color, the more color/depth there is on the rest of your face, the higher the intensity overall.

The chart is focused on orange, red, magenta, and purple hues. But any other shade from your color palette will also work (as long as you get the intensity right). So if you are a Deep Winter and want to wear midnight blue lipstick, you've got color harmony on your side!

Note: All of the shades on this chart will also work as cheek colors.

Clear Spring

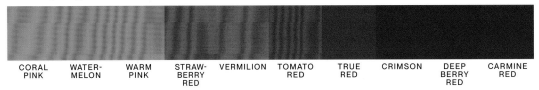

| CORAL PINK | WATER-MELON | WARM PINK | STRAW-BERRY RED | VERMILION | TOMATO RED | TRUE RED | CRIMSON | DEEP BERRY RED | CARMINE RED |

True Spring

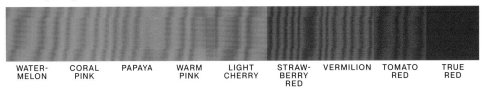

| WATER-MELON | CORAL PINK | PAPAYA | WARM PINK | LIGHT CHERRY | STRAW-BERRY RED | VERMILION | TOMATO RED | TRUE RED |

Light Spring

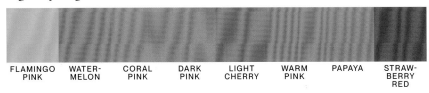

| FLAMINGO PINK | WATER-MELON | CORAL PINK | DARK PINK | LIGHT CHERRY | WARM PINK | PAPAYA | STRAW-BERRY RED |

Light Summer

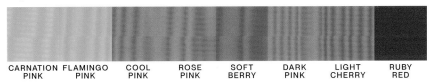

| CARNATION PINK | FLAMINGO PINK | COOL PINK | ROSE PINK | SOFT BERRY | DARK PINK | LIGHT CHERRY | RUBY RED |

True Summer

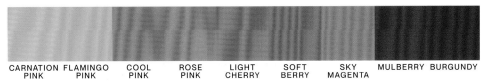

| CARNATION PINK | FLAMINGO PINK | COOL PINK | ROSE PINK | LIGHT CHERRY | SOFT BERRY | SKY MAGENTA | MULBERRY | BURGUNDY |

Soft Summer

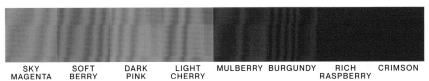

| SKY MAGENTA | SOFT BERRY | DARK PINK | LIGHT CHERRY | MULBERRY | BURGUNDY | RICH RASPBERRY | CRIMSON |

Soft Autumn

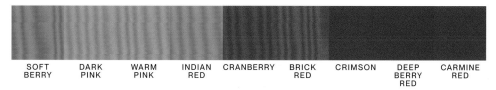

| SOFT BERRY | DARK PINK | WARM PINK | INDIAN RED | CRANBERRY | BRICK RED | CRIMSON | DEEP BERRY RED | CARMINE RED |

True Autumn

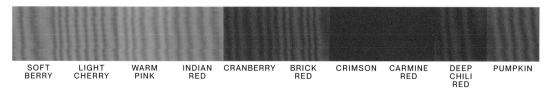

| SOFT BERRY | LIGHT CHERRY | WARM PINK | INDIAN RED | CRANBERRY | BRICK RED | CRIMSON | CARMINE RED | DEEP CHILI RED | PUMPKIN |

Deep Autumn

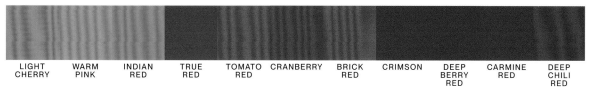

| LIGHT CHERRY | WARM PINK | INDIAN RED | TRUE RED | TOMATO RED | CRANBERRY | BRICK RED | CRIMSON | DEEP BERRY RED | CARMINE RED | DEEP CHILI RED |

Deep Winter

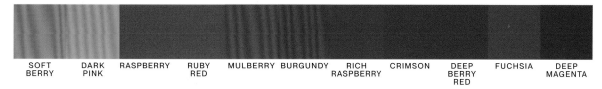

| SOFT BERRY | DARK PINK | RASPBERRY | RUBY RED | MULBERRY | BURGUNDY | RICH RASPBERRY | CRIMSON | DEEP BERRY RED | FUCHSIA | DEEP MAGENTA |

True Winter

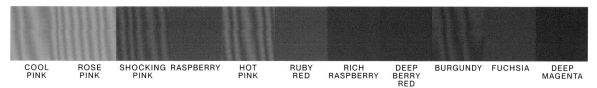

| COOL PINK | ROSE PINK | SHOCKING PINK | RASPBERRY | HOT PINK | RUBY RED | RICH RASPBERRY | DEEP BERRY RED | BURGUNDY | FUCHSIA | DEEP MAGENTA |

Clear Winter

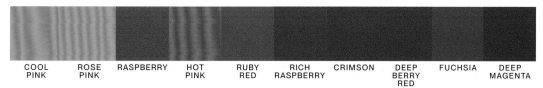

| COOL PINK | ROSE PINK | RASPBERRY | HOT PINK | RUBY RED | RICH RASPBERRY | CRIMSON | DEEP BERRY RED | FUCHSIA | DEEP MAGENTA |

Conclusion

How to start implementing your colors

You have figured out your season and explored your best colors. You know which color genres work well with your coloring, which undertones harmonize with your complexion, and how much contrast you can pull off when it comes to your hair and makeup.

What you do with this information is up to you. You likely have mixed feelings about your season's color palette: you love some colors and are excited to wear them; others, not so much. Then there are the colors you currently wear in your clothes, accessories, makeup, and hair, some of which may not be in your palette. Use these questions to take stock:

☐ Which colors from my palette do I already wear regularly?

☐ Which colors from my palette do I own (as clothes, accessories, or makeup) and want to wear more often?

☐ Which colors would I like to wear but don't own any items of?

☐ Which colors from my palette do I *not* want to wear?

☐ Which colors and items do I wear regularly that *don't* harmonize with my coloring? Do I want to keep wearing them or replace them?

Remember: Your color harmony won't be impacted by a shade that sits farther from your face, or by smaller, less harmonious color doses, such as earrings or a detail on your top. Color harmony is also not mandatory. Your taste and aesthetic always come first. There is no reason to stop wearing your favorite colors. Your goal is not to curate a closet of clothes that fits your color season perfectly—it's to wear what feels good.

Acknowledgments

Thank you to all of our gorgeous models:

Tordis Adrian, Rachel Agmase, Caroline Alexander, Yvonne Sonyaa App, Arianna, Diane Bödrich, Sarah Bunk, Zara Aylin Çelik, Theresa Deichert, Diana Dufke-Vargas, Emeka Ene, Iason Georgakopoulos, Lena Marie Großmann, Michael Hermann, Selina Afua Holdbrook-Kuessow, Jessica Johnson, Eliza Maria Jakobsen Legg, "Zondy" Nomanzondo Marth Keil, Soom Kim, Katrin Kophal, Anja Krause, Jacob Kristiansen Odgaard, Ellen Kuula Særmark-Thomsen, Rubina Labusch, Jülly Liang, Elisa Müller, Kripa Navas, Dugga Aba Pfeiffer Quardi, Camille Puget, Anastasia Reinsch, Gustavo Rocha, Signe Marie Rybjerg Andersen, Theresa Schimana, Szymon Stepniak, Tori Tyurina.

Our models are wearing clothes provided by Colorful Standard and Jan 'N June.

About the Author

Anuschka Rees is a Berlin-based writer and the author of *The Curated Closet* and *Beyond Beautiful.* Her books have been translated into more than twelve languages. She loves color, art, and fashion and enjoys the challenge of breaking down abstract visual concepts into practical takeaways. Her mom introduced her to color analysis as a teenager, and she spent twenty years identifying as a Light Spring. After immersing herself in color theory for *Personal Color,* she now knows she is a Light Summer.

anuschkarees.com

@anuschkarees

Index

Ten Speed Press
An imprint of the Crown Publishing Group
A division of Penguin Random House LLC
1745 Broadway
New York, NY 10019
tenspeed.com
penguinrandomhouse.com

Typefaces: Pangram Pangram's Neue Montreal, The Ivy Foundry's IvyPresto, Supfont's Des Montilles

Library of Congress Cataloging-in-Publication Data
Names: Rees, Anuschka, author.
LC record available at https://lccn.loc.gov/2024039588
LC ebook record available at https://lccn.loc.gov/2024039589

Trade Paperback ISBN: 978-0-593-83621-7
Ebook ISBN: 978-0-593-83622-4

Manufactured in China

Editor: Kaitlin Ketchum | Production editor: Terry Deal | Editorial assistant: Kausaur Fahimuddin
Designer: Annie Marino | Production designer: Faith Hague | Production and prepress color manager: Kim Tyner
Photography: Anna Rose | Wardrobe: Ronja Stuckn | Digitech: Szymon Stepniak | Production assistant: Signe Marie Rybjerg Andersen | Hair and makeup: Seraphine Boateng and Sydney Raab
Models: Tordis Adrian, Rachel Agmase, Caroline Alexander, Dorte Rybjerg Andersen, Signe Marie Rybjerg Andersen, Yvonne Sonyaa App, Okkar Aung, Arianna, Diane Bödrich, Sarah Bunk, Zara Aylin Çelik, Theresa Deichert, Sarah Delling, Diana Dufke-Vargas, Emeka Ene, Alexander Gatos, Iason Georgakopoulos, Graciela González de la Fuente, Lena Marie Großmann, Amin Abd El Halim, Michael Hermann, Selina Afua Holdbrook-Kuessow, Jessica Johnson, Aristos Karabelas, "Zondy" Nomanzondo Marth Keil, Soom Kim, Katrin Kophal, Anja Krause, Rubina Labusch, Eliza Maria Jakobsen Legg, Jülly Liang, Nae Lienshöft, Elisa Müller, Kripa Navas, Malcolm Ndiaye, Jacob Kristiansen Odgaard, Rohit Patel, Camille Puget, Dugga Aba Pfeiffer Quardi, Sarah Reichhardt, Anastasia Reinsch, Gustavo Rocha, Ellen Kuula Særmark-Thomsen, Theresa Schimana, Szymon Stepniak, Tori Tyurina, Michelle Ying Zhang.
Copy editor: Julie Ehlers | Proofreaders: Tracy R. Lynch, Daina Penikas, and Ann Roberts
Indexer: Elise Hess | Publicist: Kristin Casemore | Marketer: Andrea Portanova

10 9 8 7 6 5 4 3 2 1

First Edition

The authorized representative in the EU for product safety and compliance is Penguin Random House Ireland, Morrison Chambers, 32 Nassau Street, Dublin D02 YH68, Ireland, https://eu-contact.penguin.ie.